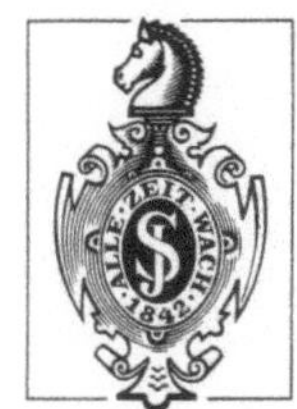

J. Møller · H. Einfeldt

# Testosterone Treatment of Cardiovascular Diseases

## Principles and Clinical Experiences

With 3 Figures and 24 Color Photographs

Springer-Verlag
Berlin Heidelberg New York Tokyo 1984

Jens Møller
President of the European Organization
for the Control of Circulatory Diseases (EOCCD)
Store Kongensgade 36
DK-1264 Copenhagen K

Helge Einfeldt
Krankenhaus St. Georg
Lohmühlenstraße 5
D-2000 Hamburg 1

ISBN-13: 978-3-642-61746-1        e-ISBN-13: 978-3-642-61744-7
DOI: 10.1007/978-3-642-61744-7

Library of Congress Cataloging in Publication Data.

Møller, J. (Jens), 1914. Testosterone treatment of cardiovascular diseases. Bibliography: p. Includes index.
1. Testosterone Therapeutic use. 2. Cardiovascular system Diseases Treatment. 3. Hormonic therapy.
I. Einfeldt, H. (Helge), 1941–. II. Title. [DNLM: 1. Cardiovascular Diseases drug therapy. 2. Testosterone
therapeutic use. WG 166 M726t] RC684.T47M65    1984    616.1'061    84-10676



© by Springer-Verlag Berlin Heidelberg 1984
Softcover reprint of the hardcover 1st edition 1984



Typesetting: Brühlsche Universitätsdruckerei, Giessen
Printing: Brüder Hartmann, Berlin. Binding: Lüderitz & Bauer, Berlin
2119/3020-543210

# Preface

For many years now I have devoted much of my time to lecturing and writing on the subject of cardiovascular disease (CVD). In this book I have outlined the development of my approach to this problem. I must admit that the details of my theories have undergone continuous modification as a result of the lessons learned in treating a large number of patients, but the basic message has remained the same. I believe that the delay in the utilization of testosterone treatment for CVD has arisen from a failure by specialists in endocrinology, biochemistry, physiology, and cardiology to understand each other's point of view and therefore to effectively coordinate their clinical efforts. This is like four people starting to climb the various faces of a pyramid, unaware of each other's presence until they reach the apex. It is hoped that bringing specialists in these different disciplines together at "summit meetings" will help them discover the true nature of this disease, the cardiovascular specialist understanding the underlying lack of anabolic steroids, and the other three grasping the way in which treatment with these compounds can effectively counteract the metabolic disturbance which is the cause of CVD.

Even apart of the language barrier, writing this book has by no means been an easy task. Please consider my situation; one cannot be a cardiologist, endocrinologist, biologist, biochemist, and physiologist all in one person. This fact may open me to criticism. This is especially true since, as everybody knows, a large army of specialists has been trained to dispute, argue, quarrel, and criticize rather than to make a constructive contribution to medical science. This army will undoubtedly turn up, but I hope that my readers will not overrate their arguments, realizing that this book presents scientific evidence which will help achieve a better understanding of the problem of CVD.

Though I am still accumulating knowledge and experience, I feel that the time has now come to present the results of my efforts. Furthermore, I have been encouraged to publish my views at this time by a large number of people who have followed and supported my work with circulatory diseases from the beginning. Lately there have been such important progress within CVD research and ardent discussion of it that I do not hesitate to participate in the discussion by relating my experience based on the treatment of many patients over the years and the positive results that I have had with testosterone treatment of CVD. CVD is a topic that is very difficult deal with following the rules that ordinarily apply to scientific papers. Had I attempted to conform strictly to the rules, in my opinion much would have been lost. I have thus reported in this study on my long experience with CVD and patients suffering from it. In this connection, there is no doubt that apart from the above-mentioned army there are many who take part in the debate because they are used to entering any arena as soon as an opportunity arises, in spite of their complete lack of knowledge with regard to CVD and CVD patients.

My original intention was to keep strictly to my subject and avoid every mention of the controversies to which I have been a witness. In the meantime, however, these polemics have developed into contentions the nature of which I, as a doctor, have never experienced. I realize now that I cannot avoid being involved in these bitter discussions, although this is much against my will. The controversies covered both the factors causing CVD and the medication for it. With regard to the causes, for a long time diet has been "in". One party claims that margarine can prevent the formation of thrombi in coronary vessels and consequently cure CVD, and that butter promotes the formation of thrombi. Another party calls this postulate pure nonsense and claims that margarine is carcinogenic. Both parties can substantiate their results statistically. Recently, however, other scientists have found that thrombi in coronary vessels are not the cause of CVD, but are produced by a lack of oxygen under certain circumstances, regardless of whether butter or margarine has been eaten. With regard to medication, one pharmaceutical agent was developed, tested in multicenter trials, and reported to lower cholesterol levels, thus able to eliminate this cause of CVD. Other researchers found that the agent had fatal effects. Another substance was found to lower blood pressure, another factor in CVD, and again the magical statistics were applied. Now it has been proved that this substance can also be fatal for CVD patients.

Epidemiological trials are also carried out, but seldom appear to result in anything that helps the unfortunate patient. In my evaluation of these trials I can hardly avoid visualizing the story told by our famous Danish poet Hans Christian Andersen. The tailors, pretending to do something with their empty gestures, produced the same results in "The Emperor's New Clothes" as many researchers in these trials.

In front of me I have a book entitled *Science and Common Understanding* by Robert Oppenheimer (1960) with a foreword by Niels Bohr. This book contains the following quotation from Thomas Jefferson:

The medical world is in an even worse state than that of total ignorance. If we could free ourselves from all that we believe we know about medicine, we could start from a higher level and with a clearer view. From Hippocrates to Brown we have had nothing but a series of hypothetical systems which, in turn, have been in fashion for a while, just as hat and dress fashions, and thereafter made room for the next craze. And yet the human body, which is the object of suffering and torture because of these pseudoscientific methods, has not changed.

How well that applies to our time! Holberg, the great Danish playwright, several hundred years ago wrote the common Danish story about a young country lad, the son of a farmer, who had studied at the University of Copenhagen and learned how to dispute scientifically, a situation which has not changed much since then. He chose his dear old mother as the subject of his cleverness, in order to win the admiration of the villagers. "I can prove that you are a stone, mother!" he said. "You cannot fly, a stone cannot fly, therefore you are a stone." On hearing this the simple woman began to cry, imagining that she could feel herself becoming as heavy as a stone. Fortunately the young man was then able to convince her that she was not a stone since she could speak and a stone cannot. This is just the same as the butter and margarine story: "By debate I can prove that this substance can cure you or can prove that it can kill you."

The clinical results achieved in my clinic for cardiovascular patients in Copenhagen are by now well known in Europe, America, and Japan, and this has encouraged further research, particularly into the widespread metabolic effects of testosterone treatment. Better understanding of these processes could perhaps optimize the results of treatment by enabling regulation of dosage according to laboratory results.

Finally I am very grateful to those whose support made possible the completion of this book. I must express my appreciation of the scientific support and medical experience of Dr. Helge Einfeldt, Secretary General of the European Organization for the Control of Circulatory Diseases (EOCCD), whose assistance and enthusiastic encouragement has been instrumental.

I also greatly appreciate the support of the Danish Society for the Prevention of Circulatory Diseases *(Landsforeningen til Bekæmpelse af Kredsløbssygdomme, LBK)*, which is the most important and serious organization in Denmark dedicated to helping the unfortunate patients suffering from CVD. The managing committee of this organization has urged us to finish this book, and the members of the board have contributed to its completion with their idealistic as well as financial support. The unselfish commitment of the organization and its members has been an outstanding example to me and my associates. The LBK is deserving of our gratitude. Furthermore, I am grateful to my British secretary, Rosemary Christensen, who has spent her time and effort in helping us with the writing and translation of the many drafts of this book. Last but not least I have to emphasize my thanks to medical student Michael Lützhøft Hansen for his productive and indefatigable labor, review of the literature, and extensive clerical work.

The authors would like to thank *Dr. Friedrich Husmann* for providing the text which appears on the back cover of this book. *Dr. Husmann,* formerly Professor of endocrinology of the University of Würzburg, has spent many years specializing in internal medicine and has won international esteem for his numerous articles, books and lectures. He has done research and clinical work on the use of testosterone in the treatment of cardiovascular diseases. He is currently medical director of the Klinik am Malerwinkel in Bad Sassendorf, Federal Republic of Germany.

# Contents

# Historical Review

Having made the acquaintance of Dr. Jens Møller at his clinic in Copenhagen and seen the results of his treatment, I felt inspired to search through the medical literature to find accounts of research on testosterone and its effects on cardiovascular disease (CVD) or the parameters of CVD which had been carried out before J. Møller started his work in this field. As a result I was able to produce a report, written in German and Danish (Einfeldt 1970, 1976), containing short descriptions of the results obtained by many scientists as well as extracts from research papers.

Much of the information used in this earlier scientific work will be included in this review. It soon became clear to me that the parameters of CVD are both interrelated and interdependent, which means that they all influence CVD more or less strongly and that testosterone treatment of one will affect the others.

This book deals in particular with the life-giving and life-maintaining substance testosterone (containing the cyclopentanoperhydrophenanthrene nucleus). As early as the time of Jesus Christ, the Greeks were convinced of the existence of such a substance, which they believed to have some connection with the male sexual glands and be of vital importance to the physiology of the entire organism. Strangely enough, many hundreds of years were to pass before we, in this era, began to appreciate this fundamental fact; only recently have we begun to make an effort to find and isolate this substance. This ancient Greek idea was scientifically confirmed in 1849 by the German physiologist Arnold Berthold at the University of Göttingen, who was able to produce secondary sexual characteristics in capons by implantation of testicles from sexually mature cocks. As a matter of fact, the experiment made by Berthold led to a test of androgen activity, the so-called cock'scomb test. The increase in size of cock'scomb was used as a measure of testosterone's action.

The problem then remained as to how to obtain the hormone itself. It became clear that the concentration found in testicular tissue is extremely low. By experiment, Adolf Butenandt and Kurt Tscherning in Göttingen succeeded in extracting 15 mg crystalline androsterone from 15,000 liters of male urine in 1931. In 1934 these two scientists were able to state the chemical formula of the testosterone hormone molecule (Butenandt 1934), and in 1935 the Jugoslavian chemist Leopold Ruzicka in Zürich developed testosterone from cholesterol. Butenandt and Ruzicka received the Nobel prize for their research in 1935. At last, it had become possible to use testosterone in the treatment of patients.

It is perhaps of interest that it was, I believe, the famous Danish surgeon Thorkild Rovsing who proved, during the First World War, the positive effect of testosterone on circulatory disease. After a young man suffered a sudden and violent death, Rovsing transplanted his testicles into an old male patient with gangrene, with the result that the gangrene healed completely. The contents of this book are based on the positive effects of testosterone on circulation, a chapter in medical history begun by Rovsing in Denmark.

In 1938 W. H. Veil and O. Lippross observed positive results of testosterone treatment and even at that time pointed out the improved effect on the impaired carbohydrate metabolism of CVD patients as shown by a decrease in plasma glucose levels.

In 1939 the famous scientist Heinrich Schumann used testoviron experimentally in castrated and noncastrated male animals and found an increase in glycogene. He drew the conclusion that this finding could be of clinical importance.

In the same year Heinz Arndt showed that the condition of 17 men suffering from intermittent claudication and angina pectoris improved with treatment with testoviron; gangrene was also healed.

E. A. Edwards et al. (1939, 1941) used testosterone with such magnificent results that they will be quoted in extenso elsewhere in this book (see pp. 40–41).

In 1945 M. A. Lesser (1946) used testosterone propionate therapy in one hundred cases of angina pectoris. He wrote:

One hundred patients with angina pectoris, 92 men and eight women, ranging from 34 to 77 in age, have been treated during the last five years with testosterone propionate. Ninety-one per cent improved for periods ranging from 2 to 34 months. No appreciable improvement was noted following control injections of plain sesame oil... The amount of exercise which could be tolerated before the development of anginal attack was markedly increased under testosterone therapy.

Some years later, Charles D. Kochakian (1951) demonstrated an improvement in nitrogen balance due to testosterone. This is fundamental for appreciating the effect of testosterone on CVD.

In 1960 Isaac Vaissman et al. described the cholesterol-lowering effect of androgens.

R. L. Hazelwood and Kevin O'Brien (1961) modified glucagon-induced hyperglycemia in rats by using nortestosterone.

G. Fiegel et al. were able to show, in 1962, the positive effect of anabolic steroids on more than 2,000 CVD patients and a tendency to normalization of ECG changes, which will be referred to later.

The same year, W. Weissel (1962) described an antidiabetic effect of anabolic steroids, i.e., counteracting the effect of insulin resistance, and the improvement of retinopathy.

In 1963 J. L. Kalliomäki and P. Seppälä wrote that 22 CVD patients had been treated with testosterone for 1–5 months. In 12 cases a decrease in ECG abnormalities was observed.

In 1964 M. L. Tainter et al. presented results showing that anabolic steroids appear to have a direct effect on the diabetic state by decreasing blood sugar, lowering the insulin requirements, and restoring the reactivity in the insulin-resistant patient. In diabetic retinopathy, testosterone apparently arrested the progress of the pathologic changes in the majority of reported cases.

W. Meyer-Mölleringhof (1964) showed improvement in patients with angina pectoris after injections of testosterone.

Two years later, F. Hammer (1966) treated CVD patients and found more or less normalization of ECG abnormalities.

G.A.W. Krüger (1969) achieved positive results by using androgens on CVD patients.

In 1972 S. Gudbjarnason et al. observed an increase in adenosine triphosphate (ATP) with treating experimentally produced myocardial infarction in dogs with testosterone.

Before concluding this account of the review of the literature that I undertook before entering into cooperation with Dr. Møller, I feel that particular mention should be made of Professor F. Husmann, with whom I have had personal communication concerning this research. Professor Husmann has been a member of the EOCCD from the very beginning and has in every way been cooperative and helpful. He has described treatment of 25 patients from 28 to 63 years of age who all showed signs of hypercholesterolemia. Most of these patients showed ECG changes, i.e., ST depression, negative T wave – clinically, angina pectoris symptoms. They were treated daily with 150 mg androsterone derivate, gradually decreasing later to 75–100 mg daily. All symptoms were more or less normalized during the hormone treatment. In another trial Professor Husmann treated 75 CVD patients with androgens. Some of these also had diabetes mellitus. After a short observation period he found positive results in two-thirds of the patients. Claudication patients had longer walking distances, gangrene healed, and angina pectoris symptoms disappeared.

# Significance of Cardiovascular Disease (CVD)

H. Einfeldt's historical review makes it quite clear that the use of testosterone (anabolic steroids) in the treatment of CVD is by no means a modern idea. Nevertheless, in spite of the great interest shown in testosterone treatment of CVD, it would almost seem that the development has slowed down in this important field. There may be several reasons for this. One of them might be the Second World War; naturally enough it must have delayed possibilities for cooperation since Germany was the "cradle" of hormones, as is evident from what has been written up to now. Interest was again aroused when CVD was described universally, and particularly in America, as a new plague for mankind. Billions of dollars have been invested in the search for the cause and a method of combatting it, and statistics have been assembled which have aroused apprehension throughout the civilized world. The press has, no doubt unconsciously, overemphasized the seriousness of this disease, the danger of which is magnified in people's minds by the attention drawn to it every time a well-known person dies suddenly, presumably but not assuredly from CVD.

It must be mentioned, however, that great doubt has recently been raised as to whether this statistical level is really as high as claimed. In the United States, the Surgeon General's report (Department of Health, Education, and Welfare 1979; see also Harper 1980) stated that about 40% of the entire population will die from heart disease and approximately 80% of these deaths will occur between the ages of 65 and 100. Of the remaining 20%, probably half will have hereditary problems of lipid metabolism, diabetes, and hypertension that require comprehensive care. This leaves about 4% of the general population without readily identifiable defects who will die of heart disease before the age of 65.

A second source of doubt about the statistics was raised by Franke (1981):

Disorders of the heart and circulation increase sharply with age to become the commonest cause of death in the elderly, responsible for about one-third of all deaths in those over 65 and one-half of those over 85. The death rate from cardiovascular diseases rises exponentially with age.

These are just several examples out of many concerning statistics demonstrating the current level of CVD, high relative to other diseases. This relative increase may be due to the fact that diseases which have bacteriological etiology can be cured with antibiotics.

Although statistics or propaganda may understate or exaggerate the seriousness of a problem, CVD remains, nevertheless, a serious problem. Therefore it is quite natural that one should be particularly interested in trying to find a solution. Many people, including myself, are of the opinion that, in the effort to solve the problem posed by CVD, it has been mishandled to a degree that is almost unscientific, resulting in a waste of enormous financial resources. What I find even worse is the very unfortunate waste of time, which has been to the great detriment of the patients. A great deal could have been achieved by appreciating *the true nature of CVD* at an earlier date. One of the reasons for the continued deadlock between the various theories lies in the fact that a means of *curing* CVD has constantly been the goal. As I hope to make clear with my conception of CVD, the search for a cure for CVD means a search for the philosopher's stone of eternal life. What sense is there in looking for a nonexistent means of curing a disease which is not a disease in the accepted sense of the word?

Considering the ill-fated mistakes made up to now, testosterone treatment could be regarded as a kind of philosopher's stone, however with those limitations which nature herself imposes. Testosterone is an element essential for the existence and continuance of life. Of course, this does not only apply for testosterone, but it is appropriate to make a special point of testosterone because of its vital use as a therapeutic agent on CVD.

I might add that I have never become reconciled to the name "testosterone," which so obviously relates to testis tissue. The same applies to "prostaglandin," implying a strong relationship to the prostate gland. May I say, jokingly, that these names seem to discriminate between the sexes. More "neutral" terms would more appropriately cover the biologic effects of these hormones in the human organism.

When the people of the civilized world became so aware of this threat to their health, it was natural that it then became a social issue. As I have said, even though CVD may not be as widespread as the propaganda would have us believe, it remains a very important problem which inflicts enormous costs on society, for example, in hospital expenses and disability pensions, but above all it inflicts a great amount of human suffering.

I can only agree with the President of WHO, Dr. Halfdan Mahler, who said, as reported in the press, that in medical matters professional ability is not sufficient to achieve a goal, but determined effort and political decisiveness are also essential. The same view was expressed by a professor of medicine at a symposium in Strasbourg, when he said that I acted in the spirit of the great German clinician, Professor Virchow, by bringing this medical problem to the attention of the European Parliament. We have to approach those we have elected to rule our societies in order to secure cooperation, but let me emphasize that this does not mean that it is a political issue. Every country, just as every citizen, takes an interest in the health situation, so that such cooperation is not a matter of partisan politics.

# Establishment of EOCCD

Several years ago I found that certain members of the European Parliament took a great interest in the problem of CVD and the possibilities for effective treatment and prevention. Therefore, it was decided to hold a symposium led by a honorary committee consisting of the following members:

Mr. Georges Spenale
President of the European Parliament

Mr. Finn D. Gundelach
Member of the Commission of European Communities

Mr. Libero della Briotta
President of the Commission of Public Health
and Environment of the European Parliament

Mr. Christian Albertsen
Member of the Commission of Public Health
and Environment of the European Parliament

Mr. Pierre Pflimlin
Mayor of Strasbourg
(Former Prime Minister of France)

Since I was known as a member of the medical profession who had been concerned with the problem of CVD for many years, I was asked, together with other scientists working in this field, to talk at this meeting in Strasbourg.

The audience at this symposium, scientists and members of the European Parliament, agreed on the establishment of the European Organization for the Control of Circulatory Disease (EOCCD), the aim of which was to prevent and to fight this disease. At the constituent meeting of this organization's General Assembly on 7 April 1976, I was elected President. At that meeting I pointed out the possible benefits of physical activity for CVD prevention, and also urgently requested that research be carried out on testosterone treatment of CVD. Dr. Helge Einfeldt, who had been active in the same field for many years, was elected Secretary General.

Since 1976 the EOCCD has held symposia in London at the House of Lords (July 1977) and at the Royal College of Obstetricians and Gynecologists (June 1979), in Bonn (November 1978), in West Berlin (1982), and in Munich (1983). Several meetings have been hosted by the European Parliament in Strasbourg and Luxembourg.

Various working parties have been set up within the EOCCD to carry out special studies in the field of cardiovascular research. The EOCCD has also given financial support for scientific research in universities throughout the world, including an extensive research project, which has been running for 6 years in collaboration with the Medical Research Council (MRC) in Great Britain, to examine the role played by hormones in CVD.

# Effectiveness of Testosterone Treatment

## Testimony of Specialists

After these meetings of the EOCCD in Europe, the positive results of testosterone treatment were published in several EOCCD bulletins and evoked great interest throughout the medical world. Previously, however, the Danish Society for the Prevention of Circulatory Diseases, with some 50,000 members, had been very active. Since it felt very strongly that the unusually large practice in Copenhagen must be more convincing than the bulletins in demonstrating the effectiveness of testosterone treatment, it took the initiative of inviting leading specialists in CVD research from the whole world to witness the results of this treatment and assess the patient material. The following are samples of their reactions.

Professor William Boyd (1965) commented:
This form of hormone therapy has been in vogue in Germany for a number of years and I personally have seen in Copenhagen a remarkable demonstration of the relief afforded by these measures (hormone therapy), in some cases saving the patient from amputation and even suicide.

Dr. Malcolm Carruthers, from the Maudsley Hospital, London, wrote in his report (1980) after his sabbatical leave at my Copenhagen clinic in 1978:

Particularly impressive were the healing areas of gangrene and other regions of ischemic ulceration. Gangrene in one or several toes which, in most clinics would have been treated by immediate amputation, dramatically improved with anabolic steroids and antibiotics. The blackened, necrotic areas became dry and less infected and within a few weeks separated, leaving a clean healing surface. Perhaps the most dramatic, from the patient's point of view, was the relief of pain associated with ischemic lesions. Impaired sleep for months or years often results in severe depression or being on the brink of suicide. Relief of the limb pains and restlessness at night, as well as allowing sleep, which makes the patient feel well to the point of euphoria, reduces the associated stress which may contribute to the sympathetic predominance initiating from the maintaining lesion. Around 25% of the patients presented symptoms of coronary insufficiency, varying from angina on effort to a history of recent myocardial infarction. A further 25%, though presenting symptoms predominantly affecting the limbs, admitted to a history of chest pain on exertion, or had ECG signs of cardiac ischemia either at rest or on exertion testing. This is a further proof of the multifocal nature of arterial disease. On anabolic steroids there was routinely remission of these symptoms and normalisation of the S-T segment of the ECG was repeatedly observed.

Following their visit in 1979, a group from the Hammersmith Hospital (University of London) consisting of Consultant Endocrinologist C. F. Joplin, Consultant Vascular Surgeon C. W. Jamieson, and Professor of Cardiovascular Medicine C. P. Shillingford stated (Shillingford et al. 1980):

We were impressed by the healing of large and deeply penetrating ulcers in legs without foot pulses which we should not have expected to have healed in the normal course of events, but might have led to amputation of the limb.

Professor Shillingford was impressed by the good results achieved in spite of lack of pulsation, but I can perfectly well understand this phenomenon and will explain it very clearly in this book. On this same problem Zetterquist (1970) made the following comment:

Active training treatment for 3–4 months improved the walking tolerance in patients with intermittent claudication even in the absence of an increase in regional arterial inflow capacity, as estimated by venous occlusion plethysmography. This was explained, partly at least, by the observation of a more effective peripheral oxygen utilization in the exercising ischemic limb after than before training, indicating a regional redistribution of the available blood flow towards the active muscles.

Further, I refer to Remes's publications, which are mentioned later (pp. 20, 23).

Dr. Yarnell (1980) of the Medical Research Council stated:

At Dr. Møller's clinic in Copenhagen androgens have been used in the treatment of peripheral vascular disease for some 20 years. The clinic has an international reputation for clinical treatment. On my visit today I have seen 24 unselected patients aged from 30 to 82 years with peripheral vascular disorders who attended for follow-up. Documentary evidence was provided as to the extent of gangrene prior to treatment with anabolic steroids (usually testosterone in oil given i. m.). The results are impressive. Many patients have been spared amputation of fingers, toes or whole limbs. Many of the initial lesions occurred many years ago and most patients have remained disease-free since initial treatment. As Dr. Møller points out, such treatment cannot give eternal life, but the personal testament of these patients is that this treatment provides a radical improvement in their quality of life. For practical and ethical reasons, controlled trials of anabolic steroids in peripheral vascular disease have not been done in Denmark but we await the results of Professor Shillingsford's trials at the Hammersmith Hospital (United Kingdom) with interest. We, in the Medical Research Council's Epidemiological Unit in Cardiff, hope to further this pioneer work in peripheral disease by looking at another aspect of the atherosclerotic process, premature ischemic heart disease and its relationship to the plasma sex hormones *testosterone and estradiol.*[1]

Since Dr. Yarnell's visit to my clinic some very interesting publications have appeared about the relationship between heart disease and testosterone and estradiol. An article by Phillips et al. (1983) deals with this problem, comparing 61 men with coronary heart disease with 61 healthy men. The mean serum estradiol level was significantly higher in the subjects with coronary heart disease. This group was also found to have a higher plasma glucose level. The testosterone level correlated negatively with the blood glucose level in all subjects.

In Norway, Andersen et al. (1983) have approached the problem by studying 42 healthy middle-aged men with high risk of coronary heart disease. They found a highly significant correlation between a low ratio of serum testosterone to estradiol and delayed clot lysis. In this book we will probe further into the problem of fibrinolysis.

Professor E. Bergamini from the Istituto Di Patologia Generale, University of Pisa, stated (personal communication, 1982):

Your photographs depicting the clinical results you had by treating cardiovascular disease (CVD) with testosterone preparations are impressive. These are real facts. I understand why your pioneer work is being more and more appreciated by the clinical world and why famous pathologists and clinicians feel you are disclosing a solution to the enormous problem of CVD.

Finally I would like to quote the late Professor Sir Hans Krebs of Oxford University, with whom I have had personal contact (personal communication, 1982):

I feel that your clinical findings can stand by themselves and do not necessarily need underpinning as far as practical clinical medicine is concerned. After all, there are many methods of treatment which have no adequate biochemical foundation but are firmly based on clinical experience. I take it that you are anxious to see your clinical results and their interpretation be underpinned by biochemical concepts, bearing in mind that all physiological and pathological events have some biochemical basis.

I shall continually make use of extracts from bulletins and reports published by the EOCCD, some written by scientists and some by medical colleagues on the basis of what they have learned at my clinic. We must ignore the fact that they are repetitous for the sake of completeness.

## Case Studies

In this section several examples of the responses of patients to testosterone therapy are documented to illustrate the effectiveness of this treatment. The color photographs showing the extent of gangrene at various stages are in the Appendix.

The patient whose foot is shown in Fig. 4 informed me that his symptoms had first appeared 10 years before attending for treatment. Initially he had cold extremities and paresthesia; later claudication developed. The patient's condition then deteriorated further until the gangrenous stage. Sleeplessness and pain drove this patient to the brink of suicide, a state which often occurs. The patient presented with atrophy of the lower extremities, and the ECG showed the usual ST depression and inverted T wave. Treatment began with 250 mg testosterone enanthate three times a week, the typical therapy for men. Pain disappeared and the gangrene healed.

The female patient whose leg is shown in Fig. 5 has, like many other women, suffered pernio as a child, which disappeared after menarche. Gangrene appeared in connection with partus. Treatment was with 100 mg testosterone enanthate three times a week until the gangrene healed.

The case illustrated by Fig. 6 is very similar to that in Fig. 4 apart from the abrupt appearance of ulceration.

Figure 7 illustrates a special case in which the ulceration penetrated to the bone. After three years treatment was successful.

In the case shown in Fig. 8 the ulceration had also penetrated to the bone. It seems a miracle that we were successful in treating this patient, who is now able to lead a normal life and has resumed his occupation.

Figure 10 depicts the foot of an 85-year-old diabetic woman suffering from gangrene. In spite of her advanced age, the gangrene healed completely.

The foot shown in Fig. 11 is from a patient who developed gangrene after sympathectomy. This demonstrated the danger of interfering with the autonomic nervous system either medically or surgically.

Like Figs. 7 and 8, Fig. 12 shows the foot of a patient with gangrene which penetrated to the bone.

---

1 Emphasis – here as well as throughout the text – has been added.

# Nature of CVD

The guideline for the EOCCD's efforts has been my conception of circulatory diseases, which I do not consider to be diseases in the accepted sense as, for example, infectious diseases, which have bacteriological etiology and thus can be effectively treated and cured with antibiotics. The abnormal responses associated with CVD originate within the internal system of the organism itself; however, external conditions are undoubtedly of importance as with other illnesses. These external factors are of the greatest interest to the EOCCD, as are the direct prevention and treatment of CVD.

It is known that ageing brings with it an involution of many biologic functions resulting, if no other disease interferes, in the most final of involutions, death. In CVD a number of these functions are also impaired, but sometimes earlier in life and with more severity. Therefore, it is somewhat tempting to consider CVD as representing an *acceleration of the life processes*. Figure 1 illustrates this point.

Thus the conception of cure in CVD should be interpreted somewhat differently from that in other diseases, and if my theory can be proved correct, then cure can only mean improvement of the patient up to the point where he would have been if in "good health" but not beyond that point. This nuance of interpretation has important implications in dealing with CVD. It should not be taken to mean that CVD is "incurable" in the accepted sense of the word, for this would amount to accepting defeat without putting up a fight. Therapy, as applied to CVD patients, must primarily aim at restoring them to the normal declining pathway (line a in Fig. 1) and enabling them to lead the "normal" life which their age permits. To

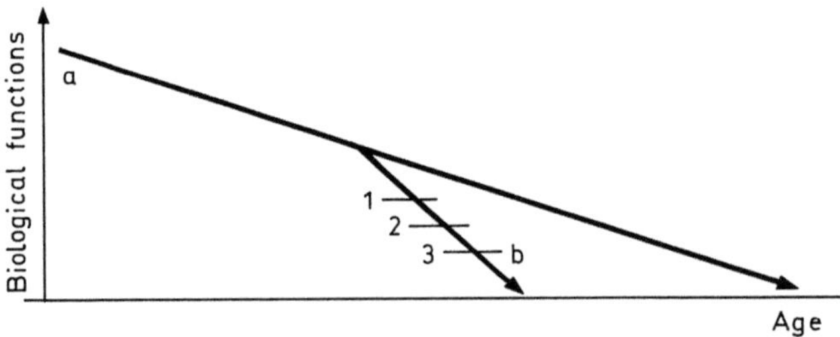


**Fig. 1.** *Line a* represents the normal deterioration of biologic functions such as stroke volume, cardiac output, arterial tension, oxygen supply, basic metabolic rate, glucose tolerance, insulin activity, and nitrogen balance as the result of ageing. (It is worth noting the influence of ageing on all the complexes of the ECG which reach their normal amplitude between the ages of 15 and 25, after which they gradually decrease.) *Line b* represents the accelerated deterioration of these functions in CVD patients. Stages: *1* intermittent claudication, angina pectoris, and ECG changes on loading; *2* pain at rest, angina pectoris, and ECG changes without loading; *3* gangrene and infarction

specifically illustrate this point, let us look more closely at CVD in the lower limbs which, according to textbooks, can be divided into three stages (line b in Fig. 1):

1. Intermittent claudication
2. Pain at rest
3. Gangrene

If the patient at stage 1 is helped back to normal walking, then the therapy has been successful. But in view of the progressive character of CVD, arresting the progress of the disease may also be regarded as a therapeutic success. For instance, stabilizing the walking distance of a patient for a considerable period means that the patient's condition does not deteriorate to stages 2 and 3. We must take into consideration the fact that everyone's circulation deteriorates sooner or later.

It seems appropriate here to mention that this normal change with age (shown by line a of Fig. 1), which is associated with a predominance of catabolic over anabolic activity, was very well described as long as a quarter of a century ago by Sobel and Marmorston (1958). I would like to quote extensively from their historic chapter here, as it clearly illustrates many of the points I am trying to make and gives a mandate for the treatment of CVD with anabolic steroids:

For this presentation let us say that ageing is a time associated biological phenomenon that is accompanied by any changes, the progression of which leads to a failure in the maintainance of vital energy and finally to death...
It is also necessary for our purpose to classify the stages of ageing as follows:
1. Growth – in which anabolic influences predominate.
2. Maturity – in which nitrogen equilibrium is attained.
3. Ageing syndrome – in which the clinical evidence of ageing becomes apparent and antianabolic influences soon predominate.

The authors then go on to discuss the role of connective tissue in the ageing process, and propose that the ratio of hexosamine to collagen (H-C) in it might be taken as a measure of biologic age.

Every cell in the body except those floating free in the blood stream is dependent upon the connective tissue for contact with its external environment. It is through the connective tissue that oxygen and nutrients reach the cells and by way of this medium that waste products are removed. The decrease in the H/C implies that the fibrillar density has increased. Accordingly, the theory has been proposed that the increase in fibrillar density may interfere with the rate of metabolic exchange that is necessary for the maintainance of vital cellular energies and functions. This may cause or condition the aging process...
It is now opportune to give attention to certain events of the aging syndrome in the human. "It is commonly accepted that as we grow old we wither away; that is, we lose flesh and become dry and cadaverous." It is also generally accepted that this major manifestation of the aging syndrome is associated with an extensive loss of body protein...
The intuitive association of the aging syndrome and its disturbed protein metabolism with the loss of *gonadal activity* is the basic precept which led to the establishment of endocrinology as a science. This concept was the background upon which Kochakian and Murlin demonstrated that androgens can cause the retention of nitrogen in castrated dogs. Now a voluminous literature exists which ascribes an anabolic activity to androgens and estrogens under certain circumstances. Since adrenals are a major source of androgenic materials as well as the anabolic steroids, it is well to inquire if the causes of disturbances in protein metabolism may be due to alterations in their secretory activity...
The fact that the excretion of *androgens and ketosteroids diminishes with age* is well documented by numerous investigators. This is particularly true of those steroids of the ll-deoxy group. In their extensive series of studies; Pincus and co-workers have pointed out that the

excretion of urinary corticoids does not diminish as rapidly with time. These observations have been confirmed in a study of the excretion of urinary steroids and corticoids by post-menopausal women. The excretion of ketosteroids was reduced with advancing age. It is of interest that women who had been chronically ill from a variety of disorders or who had suffered a severe intermittent illness in the form of *myocardial infarction* excreted less ketosteroids at every age level. The excretion of corticoids also fell with age in normal women. In younger patients the excretion was considerably lower than normal, but this difference tended to disappear with time. Calculation of the ratio of corticoids to ketosteroids (Co/K) revealed the expected finding that *this ratio increased with time*. It was considerably elevated in the patients...
Following the administration of cortisone to the rat, it was observed that decrease in hexosamine content of both skin and femurs was statistically significant. This was not the case with collagen, however. Consequently a reduction in H/C was produced. Similar reductions were observed in H/C of aorta, sternum, lungs, and trachea. Following discontinuation of cortisone treatment, partial or complete recovery of H/C ensued.
Pincus (1958) summarizes his extensive investigations with the statement that ageing and certain chronic stress conditions tend to diminish the output of certain urinary steroids. The simple conclusion would be that in aged persons the decrement is the effect of the cumulative stresses of living. In states of chronic stress this effect is telescoped...
If the age-associated alterations in the excretory pattern of urinary corticoids and ketosteroids reflect changes in the hormonal balance of antianabolic adrenal steroids and the anabolic androgens, it would be expected that as this disturbance progresses more and more, changes in the connective tissue which are induced by cortisone, as reported above, would be produced.

Finally, the authors suggest that a disturbance in connective tissue composition may increase susceptibility to arteriosclerosis or, as it is today called, CVD [Winter (1965) demonstrates that testosterone improves fibrinolytic activity].

My line of action has been to study the medical literature and to contact those scientists who are and have been concerned with normal and altered metabolism on a cellular level. I have attempted to establish whether the metabolic changes seen in CVD can be counteracted by testosterone administration, by physical training, or by both. It is not for me or the EOCCD to judge the quality of these publications; rather, we submit them for scientific discussion and feedback. Nevertheless, the publications generate considerable evidence to support the results observed with testosterone therapy. They favor the theory, supported by modern endocrinology, physiology, biology, and cardiology, that CVD must be considered to be the result of a disordered metabolism within the cell. While one remains powerless to alter the natural progress of life, the administration of testosterone makes it possible to intervene in cases where this progress has become accelerated. *Use of testosterone can improve the status of an afflicted circulatory system and has saved thousands of patients from amputation and disability; it has consequently saved many lives.*

In the following pages I shall refer to the theories developed by Kraus and Raab in *Krankheiten durch Bewegungsmangel* (1964) and many articles written since 1948 even though I am aware that their contribution has been the object of a certain amount of criticism. But he who critizes today will undoubtedly be criticized himself tomorrow.

We must always appreciate the fact that previous achievement is precisely the foundation upon which further development is built and never forget the conditions under which scientific results were achieved in the past. We should feel admiration for our predecessors in science who achieved so much without the benefit of electron microscopes, isotopes, and present-day laboratory technology. It seems grossly unfair to attack deceased scientists or any others who are not in a position to defend themselves, or the experiments which formed the basis of their publications. I tend to think that the efforts of early researchers, based on true scientific reasoning, far outshine modern technological achievement. I would like to illustrate this by referring to the book *De Motu Cordis*, published by William Harvey in 1628 (cited in Green 1976). In this treatise, Harvey put forward the experimental evidence that led him to the conclusion that blood circulates through the body. His experimental observations were so exhaustive and his reasoning so sound that very little evidence could be added today. Harvey stated: "Blood circulates, sometimes rapidly, sometimes slowly, according to temperament, age etc. of the individual, external or internal causes, normal or abnormal factors, sleep, rest, exercise, mental state and such like." Some of these factors concerning the action of the heart and the circulation of blood will now be considered in the light of current knowledge.

# Factors Affecting the Heart and Blood Circulation

Life processes advance and develop unpredictably and cannot be made the object of routine laboratory evaluation. The effects of antianabolic influences are so obvious, however, that anyone can see them in daily life. I have, for example, told my assistants that they need only watch pedestrians on the street to acquire a fundamental study of the function of circulation. A young boy crossing the street bounces over like a rubber ball. He functions like a small modern automobile, light in relationship to his powerful "engine", which ensures swift acceleration. In contrast, the adult does not have the same ability to accelerate and must evaluate the situation accordingly. Finally, the retiree knows that he cannot sprint as he did in his youth and so, consciously or unconsciously, adjusts his tempo to suit the occasion. If he exerts himself beyond his limit, the result is dyspnea and hypoxia with increased pulse rate, which might be fatal. Circulation becomes less effective as soon as one grows out of childhood. Trained athletes have attempted to copy exactly the movements of active children at play, but the athletes have had to give up. One important reason was mentioned by Steffney (1983) in the Danish newspaper *Politiken*; he stated that "on average an 11-year-old child weighs 42 kg and has a heart volume of 442 cc. The 16-year-old weighs 72 kg but only has a heart volume of 540 cc."

Let us look at this situation from a physiological point of view. The equation *heart rate × stroke volume = cardiac output* means that decreasing stroke volume results in increasing heart rate, in order to maintain adequate cardiac output. As Franke (1981) recently noted, "The really fundamental change affecting the heart and circulatory system over the course of its biological existence is the general decline in its capacity to adapt to physical exertion as age increases. Accordingly, the stroke and minute volumes and the maximal oxygen uptake – which provide a measure of the physical reserve – all decline after the thirtieth year of life."

An increase in heart rate is brought about by an increase in the production of catecholamines. If stroke volume decreases, sympathetic dominance must develop in order to maintain cardiac output. Overproduction of catecholamines can go so far as to become toxic to cells because the amount of oxygen available to cells may be insufficient to meet the metabolic requirements, leading to a shift toward anaerobic metabolism. Stimulated by adenyl cyclase, catecholamines activate phosphorylase in the liver and skeletal muscles. Blood glucose and lactic acid levels subsequently rise, with a decrease in pH and catastrophic drops in tissue ATP levels leading to cellular necrosis (e.g., gangrene and infarction). By treatment with testosterone we are able to counteract the effect of catecholamines. In accordance with the equation for cardiac output, this means an increase in stroke volume and an improvement of circulation.

## Catecholamines

More recent investigations raise the possibility that CVD is not always caused by thrombosis in the vessel walls. The literature indicates that thrombosis arises from the same circumstances as infarction and gangrene and has its origin in disturbed metabolism in the cell. Reports suggest that thrombosis can be found in vessels even in early childhood but without producing clinical symptoms. Similarly, the literature indicates that atheromatous changes in vessels are not always associated with an area of myocardial infarction. Pathological studies of such an area have shown an accumulation of catecholamines in the myocardium (Raab 1972 b, p. 710).

It is encouraging to read in the latest edition of *Goodmann and Gilman's The Pharmacological Basis of Therapeutics* (Gilman et al. 1980) that "large or repeated doses of catecholamines given to experimental animals lead to damage to arterial walls and myocardium so severe as to cause the appearance of necrotic areas indistinguishable in the heart from myocardial infarcts." Goodman and Gilman mention that the administration of calcium antagonists gives substantial protection against this damage (see also Detweiler 1979).

In this connection I should like to mention my good friend and colleague, the late Professor William Boyd, who was admired by students throughout the world for his outstanding textbooks on pathology. Even without access to the latest technical aids, he wrote in *Pathology for the Physician* (1965, p. 104) that: "The vessels are not merely passive tubes. The electon microscope has revealed a metabolic machinery capable of great activity which burns sugar, consumes oxygen and liberates carbon dioxide." It is not surprising that physicians are amazed when colleagues believe that, in the treatment of CVD, they can replace arteries with "merely passive tubes," i.e., inert plastic pipes.

The reasons for the dubious and (often) disastrous results of such treatment deserves further elaboration. I will begin by looking at the young embryo. The development of the blood vessels takes place first in the wall of the yolk sac and in the body stalk, but it also occurs later in the mesenchyme of the embryo. On the wall of the yolk sac the mesenchyme cells which are the rudiments of the blood vascular system become definitely spherical and their nuclei become relatively large. At the same time they are aggregated together into rounded patches called blood islands. As soon as the cells have attained their distinctive appearance they are known as angioblasts, and *from them are derived both the endothelial walls of the blood-vessels and blood corpuscles.* According to one view the peripheral angioblasts become endothelial cells and those more centrally situated are the ancestors of all blood corpuscles. Therefore we can hardly expect blood, having the same origin as the vessel endothelium and being anatomically, biologically and biochemically interrelated with it, to run through synthetic pipes as any inorganic liquid. I must, of course, admit that the walls of a plastic artery cannot suffer hypoxia and form thrombi in this way or from butter consumption.

Let us not forget that the decisive role in blood circulation is played by the capillaries. This is where the uptake of oxygen and nutrition and the discharge of $CO_2$ and other waste products take place. At rest, on average one hundred capillaries per $mm^2$ are open. This number may increase to 3,000 (open capillaries per $mm^2$)

during physical activity. The blood flow depends on the arterioles, which are constricted at rest and dilated during activity. The metabolic waste products and the lowering of pH due to increased metabolism cause an increased number of open capillaries, but what is most important is that the vascular system is an ingenious mechanism controlled by nervous impulses. The contractility is controlled by the autonomic nervous system in connection with the pressure-sensitive nerves. Together they form a unity, one part of the vascular system being dependent on and interdependent with the other parts. Replacement of one part of this system with inert plastic pipes disrupts this unity and shows a lack of biological insight. Have vascular surgeons ignored the fundamental anatomy and physiology of the vascular system when performing such drastic operations with their often fatal results? Please note the text accompanying Fig. 2 where I explain the improvement in oxygen supply resulting from testosterone treatment by means of an increased hexosamine-collagen ratio. My claim to be able to help almost all patients suffering from claudication is true. There are a few patients who wish to discontinue treatment since their overoptimistic expectations have not been fulfilled rapidly enough. This is precisely the category of patients who are chosen for this type of operation. No one can blame me for not being able to understand why testosterone treatment is not used since the ailment caused by the occlusion of arteries is demonstrably improved and kept under control by the fibrinolytic activity of testosterone. Here we also find an explanation for the ability of testosterone to produce such positive results in so many gangrenous patients in spite of the complete lack of pulsation of the dorsal artery of the foot, which Professor Shillingford and colleagues found so remarkable.

Sympathetic dominance of the autonomic nervous system is the physiological reaction commonly seen in response to stress; it can be provoked physically and mentally at any time, regardless of age. In an effort to shed light to the changes in metabolism which occur in response to sympathetic dominance, consider a situation where a marked physiological reaction to stress occurs. An appropriate example is a surgical operation, which produces metabolic and endocrine changes according to the length and seriousness of the operation. The endocrine responses include an increase in plasma cortisone and catecholamines, and a decrease in testosterone. Glucose tolerance is reduced and a negative nitrogen balance develops together with increased levels of free fatty acids. There is a substantial amount of literature on this subject (see, for instance, Hume et al. 1962; Nikki et al. 1972; Oyama et al. 1972; Allison 1969).

Here I feel like quoting the abstract from an article by Damber and Janson, entitled "The Effects of LH, Adrenaline and Noradrenaline on Testicular Blood Flow and Plasma Testosterone Concentrations in Anaesthetized Rats" (1978):

The acute effects of a 20-min constant rate intra-arterial infusion of LH and catecholamines on testicular blood flow and plasma testosterone concentration were examined in sodium pentobartitone anaesthetized rats. Ovine LH (2.5 g/min) elicited a 6-fold increase in testosterone concentration and a significant decrease of testicular vascular resistance. Noradrenaline and adrenaline (0.4 g/min) caused significant depressions in the plasma testosterone levels. The catecholamines induced no absolute changes in testicular blood flow, but noradrenaline caused an increase in testicular vascular resistance. The absence of changes in absolute values of testicular blood flow in the present study clearly indicates other depressive effects on testosterone secretion rather than simple vasoconstriction.

When a patient has regained conciousness after an operation, all the metabolic changes caused by operational stress are gradually reversed, normal levels being achieved due to physiological homeostasis. That is to say, a rebound anabolic process compensates for sympathetic dominance. This homeostatic process can be speeded up by administering anabolic steroids to the patient, a method used to accelerate the postoperative anabolic phase (see Tweedle et al. 1973). Patients are encouraged to accelerate the recovery process further by getting up and moving around; the relationship between physical activity and testosterone production will be discussed below.

Postoperative metabolic changes are very similar to those observed in CVD, which are described as a result of sympathetic dominance and a reaction to stress. The literature indicates that all of these metabolic changes are interrelated and interdependent and that testosterone and physical activity can each reverse these effects. We are all, of course, subject to increases in catecholamines (stress) which cause short periods of anaerobic metabolism in our daily lives. Scattered microscopic necrosis is often found in cardiac muscle on autopsy, even in very young people. Such minor necrosis had not given rise to clinical symptoms because of the normal homeostatic anabolic rebound effect. We repeat that a review of the literature leads to the conclusion that hypoxia and the related anaerobic metabolism are the root of CVD. As mentioned previously, this results in impaired carbohydrate metabolism, a lowering of pH, and a drop in tissue ATP, leading to cellular necrosis. As these are the same metabolic changes which may give rise to thrombosis, the origin of thrombosis may be the same as that of infarction and gangrene. In other words, these three may be distinct products not necessarily having any interrelationship. The relationship of arterial thrombosis to myocardial infarction indicates that some thrombi may follow, rather than precede, myocardial infarction.

This view has found support in numerous articles; I would like to quote from two of them. David Short wrote in an article entitled "The Great Circulatory Paradox" (1977) that:

*An appreciation of the role of factors other than atheroma in the aetiology of infarction is essential for rational prevention and treatment*... First there is the claim that in many cases of myocardial infarction the thrombus is younger than the infarct and therefore *a consequence rather than the cause of it*. This claim received strong support from a study in which fibrinogen labelled with radioactive iodine was injected into patients shortly after the onset of pain of myocardial infarction and the coronary arteries examined for radioactivity in those who died. In many of the cases studied the occlusive thrombus was found to be radioactive, suggesting that the thrombus was laid down after the onset of infarction [on this point see also Erlich and Shinohara 1964]... Coronary atherosclerosis is very common in adult life, and the severest degrees are often seen in people without any history of cardiac disability or evidence of either old or recent myocardial infarction... Experimentally, myocardial infarction has been reported after excessive exercise in untrained animals with healthy coronary arteries. Clinically, it is by no means rare for myocardial infarction to be precipitated by an outburst of *intense anger* or severe exertion, especially if this is sudden and relentless.

I describe such excessive exercise as "dysstress," which will be explained later (see p. 23).

I am of the same opinion as David Short that "an appreciation of the role of factors other than atheroma in the aetiology of infarction is essential for rational prevention and treatment." The press and medical journals have repeatedly published articles claiming that arteries are pipes which get sooted up due to butter consumption and can be cleared by pipe cleaners of margarine. This theory does not have anything to do with the "prevention and treatment" of CVD. The same sceptical attitude is shared by Erlich and Shinohara (1964), who wrote that there is a "relationship of arterial thrombosis to myocardial infarction" and considered "the possibility that some thrombi may follow rather than precede myocardial necrosis."

## Impaired Carbohydrate Metabolism

In the following we will probe to the very roots of CVD, which according to my theories is caused by *anaerobic metabolism resulting in impaired carbohydrate metabolism*. At the same time we must again refer to the fact that this anaerobic metabolism is caused by an overproduction of catecholamines. For example, as mentioned above, two of the consequences of operations are increased plasma cortisol and overproduction of catecholamines. It should be noted, however, that at the same time there is a *reduction of testosterone production and a decrease in glucose tolerance.* (The testosterone level correlates negatively with blood glucose, as we have frequently observed.)

The surgical stress findings mimic the metabolic changes found in CVD. According to Wagner et al. (1975):

Disturbances of carbohydrate and lipid metabolism in atherosclerosis are well-known facts. Therefore in this series of investigations relations between blood sugar, serum insulin, lipid metabolism and serum testosterone should be studied. – Patients with myocardial infarction showed significantly higher serum levels of total lipids, total cholesterol, triglycerides, and insulin. – Blood sugar was significantly higher and serum testosterone was significantly lower in patients with myocardial infarction.

To continue with carbohydrate metabolism, which is such an essential factor of the whole problem, CVD mortality rates are twice as high in patients showing reduced glucose tolerance (Fuller et al. 1980). With reference to the relationship between gradual circulatory deterioration and ageing, including impaired carbohydrate metabolism, depicted in Fig. 1, moving down lines a and b it becomes more and more difficult to distinguish what is ageing and what is disease.

Samuel Goldstein (1978) has commented: "It has so far not proved possible to distinguish the age-related and generally established 'physiological sclerosis' with certainty from pathological arteriosclerosis."

Doyle (1983) has also described ageing:

Man, like other biological species, appears to have a genetically determined life span. That is to say that those individuals who escape accidental early death due to trauma or infection survive for a finite period of time, which has not altered appreciably since historical records have been available. The word "age" is often used to denote the passage of time which refers to chronological age. The ageing process, however, involves other factors than time alone, such as physical and mental illness, trauma, and stress which accelerate the normal ageing process. The ageing process therefore involves two main processes: time related, involutional "physiological" changes and disease or stress induced "pathological" changes. In practice it is often difficult to dissociate these two processes.

The effects of ageing on the cardiovascular system include a reduction in cardiac output, an increase in energy expenditure to given amounts of cardiac work, increased oxygen debt and an increase in peripheral vascular resistance. These anatomical and physiological changes lead to impaired tissue perfusion and nutrition adding to or accelerating the time related changes at organ level.

Franke (1981) has remarked: "Impaired carbohydrate metabolism is a result of the decreased insulin activity which develops with ageing and is of course associated with a reduction in glucose tolerance." As pointed out in the *USA Diabetes Source Book* (1969), "the incidence of latent and manifest diabetes mellitus increases with age" in the same way as manifest and latent CVD increases with age. It is also worth noting that "CVD mortality in overt diabetes is 2–6 times higher than in a non-diabetic population" (Krall 1970). It has been claimed in the literature that testosterone decreases the hyperglycemic effect of glucagon (Landon et al. 1962).

Of interest is a publication on the use of anabolic steroids in therapy of diabetic patients by Tainter et al. (1964), from which I would like to quote several important passages.

There is one aspect of the metabolic defect in diabetes, however, which has not been discussed to the same extent and which is the main interest in the present paper. This is the depletion of the protein stores in the insulin-dependent diabetic patient and his frequent negative nitrogen balance. The interrelationship of insulin and other hormones to protein metabolism has been summarized thoroughly recently by Korner and Manchester. They state that uncontrolled diabetes is accompanied by a loss of body weight, depletion of tissue protein, and an increase in the rate of nitrogen excretion. This tissue wastage can be overcome by insulin, although this hormone has little effect on the nitrogen balance in non-diabetic animals or patients. The insulin has a direct action on tissues which leads to increased uptake of amino acids and their incorporation into new formed protein…
It has been generally accepted, according to Korner and Manchester, that the exaggerated loss of nitrogen shown by the experimentally produced insulin-deficient animal is caused by the secretion of *corticosteroids which are not balanced by the anabolic actions of the deficient insulin. The anabolic steroids to be discussed here also antagonize the catabolic actions of cortical steroids and have an effect on blood sugar levels.* Therefore, their possible role in the management of the diabetic patients becomes a topic of interest for discussion in this paper…
Their initial observation was that administration of 30 mg methandrostelone per day for 5 days to a patient with normal blood sugar caused marked hypoglycemia with the usual accompanying symptoms…
This peripheral action of the steroid in diabetic patients has been analyzed in considerable detail by several investigators. Weissel reported that in 3 of his 7 diabetic patients nandrolone phenpropionate had a definite antidiabetic action. He observed that it increased the response to insulin, overcame insulin resistance, relieved acidosis and produced a gain in weight. The general improvement in nutritional state was accompanied by favorable changes in the pathological effects present in the kidney and retina…
Based on investigational data, the synthetic anabolic steroids appear to have a direct action on the diabetic state by reducing blood sugar, lowering the insulin requirements, restoring reactivity in the insulin-resistant patient, and improving the general condition through better appetite, weight gains and sense of well-being. In diabetic retinopathy they apparently have *arrested* the progress of the pathological changes in the majority of reported cases. It has been postulated that this is due to the protein anabolic effects which offset the tissue protein deprivation which is characteristic of diabetes. However, since the anabolic steroid can effect both carbohydrate and protein metabolism at the cellular level, there are various other possible mechanisms by which they might favorably affect diabetic retinopathy.

My theories are an attempt to elucidate the connection between CVD and anaerobic metabolism – which, as I have said, is analogous to impaired carbohydrate metabolism – as well as the normalizing effect of testosterone on this patho-logical condition. Support for my theories has come from numerous sources. Al-banese has reported (1965): "The application of anabolic steroids appears to have direct action on the diabetic state by reducing blood sugar, lowering the insulin requirements, [and] restoring activity in the insulin-resistant patient." Talaat et al. (1957) have also reported an investigation of "the effect of repeated intra-muscular injections of testosterone propionate on the glucose tolerance and on the insulin sensitivity curves of 16 health adult male subjects." According to their results, "glucose tolerance curves were statistically altered by testosterone. There was a significant increase in the sensitivity to insulin after treatment with testos-terone." It is also worth mentioning the work of Dr. Gall of Würzburg Univer-sity, who announced in Strasbourg in June 1975 that healthy individuals taking orally active androgens showed reduced fasting blood sugar levels. It comes as no surprise, therefore, that CVD patients being treated with heavy doses of testoster-one are often advised to carry glucose tablets in case of hypoglycemia. Similarly, experience shows that diabetic patients easily succumb to insulin shock when treated with testosterone.

## Physical Activity and Stress

Physical activity is another very important factor in the control of CVD. The first precaution taught to medical students concerning the administration of insulin to diabetic patients is that the dosage must be regulated according to the activity of the patient. The more active, the smaller the dose.

Remes et al. (1979), for example, concluded from their study "that *physical train-ing can increase endogenous androgen production and that it is partly by this mech-anism that the beneficial effects of training may be achieved.*" According to this study, physical activity causes an increase in androgen production, which in turn has a positive effect on carbohydrate metabolism because of an increased re-sponse to insulin.

Let us now look at the problem from the opposite viewpoint. According to Rose et al. (1969), stress leads to an inhibition of testosterone secretion. In their article entitled "Androgen Responses to Stress" they write:

The excretion of testosterone, epitestosterone, androsterone, and etiocholanolone was measured in 27 recruits during the first month of basic combat training, in seven Special Forces personnel anticipating an immiment attack in Vietnam and in a comparison group of 12 men engaged in routine daily activities. There are several lines of evidence which in-dicate that many individuals responded to the potential threat or challenge of these situations with an inhibition of testosterone secretion.

This is an example of dysstress affecting testosterone production due to an over-production of catecholamines (see p. 23).

Aakvaag et al. (1978) have actually seen the problem in its entirety. They observed that, during a period of prolonged stress, testosterone production in young men fell initially (dysstress) and that the cortisol level rose; this was later followed by increased testosterone production (eustress), which rose to a higher level than be-fore the stress loading period. "The effect of stress on plasma testosterone can be seen. A gradual and rapid drop was observed from a mean value of 5.6 ng/ml $\pm$ 1.4 to a nadir of 0.9 ng/ml $\pm$ 0.5 on day 5. After 6 h sleep (day 6) the mean value of 1.8 ng/ml $\pm$ 0.4 was already significantly higher than on day 5 ($P < 0.001$). The level observed on day 12, 6.9 ng/ml $\pm$ 1.8, was significantly higher than on day 1 ($P < 0.05$)."

Under normal conditions a balance is maintained between plasma cortisol and insulin. When there is an increase in cortisol concentration, there is increased resistance to insulin and a consequent rise in plasma glucose (Keele and Neil 1961, p. 458). During dysstress there is an increased concentration of cortisol which results in increased resistance to insulin with an impairment of carbohydrate metabolism; in other words, there is a deterioration of circulation. This is a very important point when talking about excessive physical activity, for instance in connection with athletes being pushed to the point of exhaustion during competition. Let me emphasize here, as I shall do again, that this is a form of dysstress which very often may have serious consequences on the circulation and result in infarction and death.

This relationship can also be described in another way. When the normal production of catecholamines is increased to an excessively high level, the myocardial cells will subsequently demand more oxygen for their metabolic requirements than is available. The consequence is a shift toward anaerobic metabolism, with a dangerous drop in ATP production. The lactate and $H^+$ concentration will rise, thereby inactivating the enzymes and causing irreversible cellular damage – necrosis. This dangerous passage from eustress to dysstress can happen to any of us but is especially dangerous with increasing age. Here it is appropriate to mention that Raab (1949) has described a fourfold increase in catecholamine concentration in the heart from youth to old age, emphasizing the deterioration of circulation with advancing age, in agreement with line a in Fig. 1. The subject has also been treated by Starnes et al. (1981).

**Testosterone and Physical Training**

I will try to show in general terms the relationship between the positive effect of testosterone and the positive effect of physical training on the circulation. Efficient functioning of the striated muscles is of the utmost importance to all life-maintaining processes, and the skeletal muscles have a decisive influence on circulation. Physical activity, as mentioned, causes a release of catecholamines which affect myocardial function. If the exertion is excessive, hypoxia of the tissues can arise from the extreme oxygen demand. If physical activity is limited to avoid hypoxia, then both skeletal and cardiac muscles can be exercised in a beneficial way by increasing the oxygen-saving vagal tone with an increase in stroke volume.

It is thus possible to exercise the heart to a point where it can hold more than twice as much blood and is able to pump this entire volume instantaneously into the circulation. In addition, the exercised striated muscle is capable of more efficiently extracting oxygen from the blood, as illustrated by increased arteriovenous oxygen difference. Remes et al. (1979) observed, in their study of long-term physical training, that during a 6-month period there was a 16% increase in the estimated maximal oxygen uptake, which favors aerobic metabolism. These are the reasons that athletes exhibit lower heart rates, greater end-systolic ventricular volumes, and greater volumes at rest than nonathletes. Consequently, athletes are able to increase cardiac output without increasing their heart rates as much as their nonathletic counterparts. Increased oxygen demand, caused by catecholamines, produces a tendency to anaerobic metabolism as can be seen on an ECG in the familiar changes in ST depression and the flattening of the T wave. Similar alterations in the ECG of a nonathlete's heart can be seen when the oxygen tension in the inspired air is reduced. This should not occur in an exercised heart. The fall in phosphocreatine and ATP levels which occurs when an exercised heart is loaded is smaller than that for an nonexercised heart. Heavy loading of an exercised heart is less likely to produce a ST depression or a flattening of the T wave which are characteristic of hypoxia. An extended diastolic rest period contributes to an improved blood and oxygen supply to the ventricles. The lactic acid level in the blood also increases with exercise, but this is much lower if the heart is exercised. If physical training is not maintained, however, higher lactate levels will result within a few weeks; this is even true for young people in good physical condition. Accompanying this is an inefficient rise in pulse rate, even at modest loading, instead of the rise in stroke volume seen in the exercised heart.

With regard to anaerobic metabolism, Okamoto et al. (1983) have made some interesting comments on the consequences of reducing the oxygen tension in inspired air. They studied "the effect of hyperoxic or hypoxic inhalation on blood lipid levels and on the development of·atherosclerosis in young male WHHL rabbits" and described their experiment as follows:

They [the rabbits] were exposed to ordinary room air containing different concentrations of oxygen: 6 animals were exposed to 40% oxygen (hyperoxia group) or 5%–10% oxygen (hypoxia group) for 5 h a day, 5 days a week for 8 weeks. Four control rabbits inhaled ordinary room air. The following results were obtained.
The severity of aortic lesions significantly decreased in the hyperoxia group...
Plasma triglycerides levels were elevated only in the hypoxia group...
Likewise, Adams and Zemplenyi found that hypoxia in aortic tissue resulted in impairment of several energy-linked enzyme activities and related this to the development of atherosclerotic changes. Thus, inhalation of low levels of oxygen may, at least in part, locally influence the process of atheroma formation in aortic tissue through alterations in tissue lipid catabolism. High oxygen inhalation may reverse the process.

It is interesting to compare these findings with the words of Professor Boyd in *Pathology for the Physician* (1965, p. 104) and to compare these Japanese findings with the new attitude to thrombosis, that namely it has the same cause as infarction, i.e., an oxygen deficiency in metabolism.

The sympathetic dominance which results from excessive physical exertion, causing hypoxia and cardiotoxicity, can also result from emotional tension at rest (see Short 1977 and discussion on page 17). Sympathetic overactivity of the latter origin involves physiological suppression of muscle activity. In this connection I would like to quote from the 10th edition of *Best and Taylor's Physiological Basis of Medical Practice* (Detweiler 1979, pp. 3–117):

Another and possibly related action of catecholamines on the heart involves calcium ions. $Ca^{++}$ is required for activation of phosphorylase, and through its action in excitation-contraction coupling probably is responsible for the inotropic action of catecholamines. When applied to cardiac muscle the catecholamines both increase the permeability of the cell membrane to extracellular $Ca^{++}$, and mobilize calcium ions from intracellular stores in the sarcoplasmic reticulum. Cyclic AMP is the intermediary of this latter calcium mobilization. These processes, therefore, involve two series of interrelated reactions. In the first the catɛcholamine, acting via adenyl cyclase, 3′,5′cyclic AMP, and phosphorylase b and a, promotes glycogenolysis and simultaneously mobilizes intracellular calcium stores. In the second the catecholamine meanwhile has increased cell membrane permeability to extracellular $Ca^{++}$. The overall results are the provision of energy from carbohydrate, the mobilization of calcium ions from both extra- and intracellular sites, and the positive inotropic, etc., actions on the heart.

An overproduction of catecholamines may lead to spasm in the myocardial cells (including vascular smooth muscles), which may have fatal consequences (see Weiner 1980).
The exercised heart, with increased vagal tone and sympathetic-inhibiting influence, displays a lower rest frequency, faster return to the resting state after loading, longer contraction period, and relatively small stroke volume at rest compared with during exercise. On exertion there is a large stroke volume with high productivity and no concurrent hypoxia-dependent ST depression during loading. During sympathetic overactivity, the frequency and force of the contractions are increased, but at the expense of oxygen economy. In essence, there is a reduction in the conversion of combustible energy into mechanical work (decreased efficiency). Increased vagal tone has the opposite effect of reducing pulse rate and energy consumption in relation to productivity (increased efficiency).
Accordingly, an excessive increase in sympathetic activity, from either mental or physical stress, should induce serious cardiac results involving tachycardia and arrhythmias which are detrimental to the entire circulatory system. Subsequent myocardial hypoxia can cause angina pectoris attacks and lead to degeneration of the myocardium with diffuse necrosis and finally death. *Although many unresolved problems remain concerning CVD, there is good reason to support the notion that in some cases lack of physical activity promotes CVD and that physical training may be an effective form of therapy.* After all, life is both physical and mental activity, resulting in an alternating balance between the sympathetic and the parasympathetic systems, the one being dependent on the other. This is the balance that is vital. Predominance of the one can be just as dangerous as predominance of the other. To weaken the sympathetic system by surgical intervention (sympathectomy) or by medical blocking can have fatal consequencs. I cannot warn my colleagues strongly enough against interfering with the autonomic nervous system.
"Eu-stress" is the level of stress which causes a sympathetic response leading to rebound parasympathetic activity. In daily life, this state is achieved when suitable, sensible physical activity is followed by a period of rest for relaxation and recuperation. Mental and physical exertion beyond the limit of eustress becomes "dys-stress" where the sympathetic state dominates over the parasympathetic and becomes cellulotoxic.
Concerning anaerobic metabolism, Remes et al. (1979) showed that, after 6 months of physical training, there was an increase in the total red cell volume and red cell 2,3-DPG (diphosphoglycerate) concentration. During the 6-month period the mean plasma testosterone level increased very significantly, by 21%. The mean increase was higher in the group in good condition than in that in poor condition. In the ten subjects in best condition, the mean increase was 43%, in contrast to a 13% increase in the ten subjects in worst condition. An increase on the

order of 20%–25% for the plasma concentration of the hormones studied occurred concomitantly with a significant increase in the estimated maximal oxygen uptake ($\dot{V}O_2$ max), suggesting normal adaption to increased aerobic power. Remes et al. conclude, as I noted before, "that physical training can increase endogenous androgen production and that it is partly by this mechanism that the beneficial effects of training may be achieved."

This demonstrates the similarity between the effect of physical activity and testosterone administration. To repeat the conclusion of Remes et al., one can equate physical activity with an increase in testosterone production. Consequently, testosterone must increase 2,3-DPG concentration, which has been confirmed by Ganong in his book *Review of Medical Physiology* (1975).

At this point it is appropriate to refer to a publication establishing that physical training and testosterone treatment have the same effect and confirming several aspects that have already been dealt with. This is the study by Janda et al. (1976) on "the effect of the anabolic hormone 19-nortestosterone propionate (Superanabolon Spofa) on the metabolism of chronically ischaemic (ischaemia was produced by ligature of the right common iliac artery) striated muscle (anterior tibial m.) ... in a described model in rats." The report of this research deserves to be quoted extensively because of its importance.

Administration of 19-nortestosterone propionate prevented enzymatic changes which are typical for chronic ischaemia, primarily the decrease in the activities of dehydrogenases of Krebs' cycle tricarboxylic acids (MDH, SDH). In addition, the ratio of red to white muscle fibres increased. Administration of *anabolic hormone has a similar favourable action on ischaemic muscle as training studied previously.*

Anabolic steroids are routinely used in the treatment of all states which involve a negative nitrogen balance, e.g., severe nutritional deficiencies, states following severe operations trauma, some cases of nephropathy, but also as a general support of reparative processes in a number of other diseases such as diabetic retinopathy, peptic ulcers, trophic skin ulcers, etc. (Bleha and Küchel 1967). There has also been application of these hormones in cardiology. The most well known application is the favourable effect on myocardial metabolism in potassium depletion. Administration of testosterone or other anabolic steroids can correct slight pathological changes in the ECG, improve the functional capacity of the myocardium, in some cases result in an amelioration of angina pectoris and in most cases improve the general state of well-being (Fiegel 1961; Haan 1963).

In recent years, attempts have been made to use protein-anabolic hormones to induce a muscular development in athletes involved in particularly strenuous sports such as rowing, weight lifting, etc. The results have been reported to be better than those with training alone (Johnson and O'Shea 1969).

The above applications led us to attempt to use anabolic hormones in the treatment of ischaemia of the lower extremities. The original intention was to accelerate the healing of trophic skin ulcers which can complicate advanced stages of this disease. It was shown, however, that this therapy also resulted in a decrease of subjective complaints such as claudication, pain at rest, palpation sensitivity in ischaemic muscle, and the functional capacity of the involved extremities improved.

The fact that administration of an anabolic steroid prevents the decrease in activities of MDH, SDH, and CE in ischaemic muscle in the animals shows a positive metabolic effect of these steroids. The Krebs' cycle tricarboxylic acids, involved in the function of MDH and SDH, are the richest source of ATP, necessary not only for muscular work, but also for many other metabolic reactions, including proteosynthesis, which is primarily stimulated by these anabolic hormones. *The above effect of Superanabolon ist very similar to the favourable effect of training on the metabolism of ischaemic muscle* (Janda et al. 1972; Urbanová et al. 1974), which also prevents a decrease in the activities of the dehydrogenases of the Krebs' cycle under conditions of chronic ischaemia. There is also agreement with the fact that both after training and administration of Superanabolon, there was a certain degree of morphological and functional transformation in the white zone of the ischaemic muscle; there was an increase in red muscle fibres at the expense of white in the same zone, although this transformation was less marked following anabolic hormones than following training.

It is known that testosterone may influence muscle glycogen content in animal experiments and improves glucose utilisation especially in androgen sensitive muscles – e.g. m. levator ani (Bergamini et al. 1969; Bergamini 1969), but also in other skeletal muscles in general (Leonard 1952; Talaat et al. 1958, 1964; Gillespie and Edgerton 1970).

A favourable metabolic effect of training in both normal and ischaemic muscles has also been intensively studied in recent years, e.g. training improves oxygen utilisation by working muscles of an ischaemic extremity (Zetterquist 1970; Koppelman 1973; Carlson and Pernow 1962; Pernow et al. 1973)... A number of biochemical parameters, clearly abnormal in ischaemic muscle, are improved by training (Holm et al. 1973; Gillespie and Edgerton 1970; Janda et al. 1974).

A disturbance in the synthesis of macroergic phosphates – ATP, creatine phosphate – explains some of the manifestations of ischaemic disease of the lower extremities, such as decreased functional capacity and increased rate of fatigue in the ischaemic extremity (Pernow et al. 1973). A decrease in activities of enzymes of the tricarboxylic acid cycle suggests that under conditions of chronic ischaemia this metabolic pathway is damaged, which represents a decrease in the most effective energetic use of carbohydrates and the richest source of macroergic phosphates in both muscle and other tissues. It would be logical to find a basis of the above clinical signs of ischaemic disease of the lower extremities precisely in this metabolic disturbance. The biochemical findings in ischaemic muscle following administration of anabolic steroids showed some degree of repair of metabolic processes in this tissue, and this would, to some degree, explain the clinical improvement in patients treated in the same manner.

Inspired by this and similar articles, the EOCCD has supported investigations at the Institute for Biology and Chemistry at Roskilde University Center, Denmark, concerning the effect of testosterone on enzyme activity in patients suffering from CVD. The preliminary reports show (in agreement with the article just quoted) improved activity of succinate dehydrogenase (SDH) and glucose 6-phosphate dehydrogenase. There was a relation between these findings and patients' clinical improvement.

Physical activity can decrease the production of catecholamines by training the heart to pump a greater stroke volume, thereby reducing the pulse rate and thus improving the circulation. Improved circulation means improved *aerobic* metabolism, which again means improved enzyme activity. All the anabolic processes are improved, including *testosterone* production. With regard to hormones, Stryer commented in his *Biochemistry* (1975): "Hydroxylation reactions play a very important role in the conversion of cholesterol to steroid hormones and bile salts. All of these hydroxylations require NADPH and $O_2$." This theory explains why physical activity may be used prophylactically to improve circulation which is slowly deteriorating, a situation which would not normally be recognized as a circulatory disease. A doctor would not, therefore, prescribe testosterone treatment.

I myself was curious to find out what could be achieved with physical training over a short period. Therefore I arranged for 64 hard-working shipbuilders to spend 8 days at a physical training college. These men, whose ages ranged from 24 to 67 years, were screened and trained daily for 4–5 h. Besides the physical training, which consisted of swimming, jogging, and gymnastics, they had the opportunity of playing badminton, table tennis, and billiards. Almost all were in poor physical condition, as was revealed by ECG results after exercise stress tests.

What then did we achieve? After 8 days we confirmed, among other positive factors, that there was on average a 20% decrease in cholesterol levels and a tendency to normalize blood pressure and ECG changes. It should be added that the participants were very satisfied and grateful for their improved condition; hence it follows that physical and mental well-being *are* connected.

As a final comment on the subject of physical activity, it is generally accepted that one should not, or perhaps cannot, move in the same way after the age of 30 as before. Starting with that age, the stroke volume and the amplitudes on the ECG decrease and it is considered natural to put on weight. Attempts to stay in top physical condition, regardless of age, could be considered abnormal. This is another area where the EOCCD is determined to revise accepted ideas without neglecting common sense. We do not wish to force people who feel well to take advantage of the facilities available for physical training if they are not inclined to do so.

## The Propaganda for Physical Activity

I have described the influence of the autonomic nervous system and physical training on CVD. Uninhibited and fanatical propaganda for physical training can have a negative effect on the circulation of some people by giving them a guilt complex. They are made to feel that insufficient physical activity will result in circulatory disease or death. Through the autonomic nervous system this can make exercise a strain on deficient and normal circulation. Moreover, it is scientifically senseless to postulate that physical activity can increase the length of life, which of course cannot be proved. *The beneficial effects of physical activity are highly individual.* I feel I should repeat that competition in physical activity must be strongly condemned as far as improving the circulation is concerned.

It is a fact that many people who live a normal life without excessive activity achieve a ripe old age and get through life without extraordinary impairment of their circulation. The physical activity in their normal daily lives is sufficient. One must destroy the neurosis which has overtaken large segments of the population, which for example leads people who are not in good condition to participate in races, often with death as the result. The members of the medical profession responsible for the propaganda encouraging this have shown a complete lack of understanding of the physiology of circulation. It is obvious that young people who do not exert themselves physically in their daily lives benefit from exercise. They are also producing endogenously the hormones which contribute to these beneficial results. The internal production of these hormones declines with age, setting a limit for the results of an older person. The person with reduced internal production of testosterone more easily exceeds the limit of eustress by exerting himself physically, thus achieving a state of dysstress or, in other words, anaerobic metabolism with all of its destructive effects and possibly fatal consequences. If there are facilities for physical activity, people should use them of their own free will and on their own initiative provided that the result is physical and mental well-being.

Another example of the harm that can be done by such propaganda about physical training is that our many disabled patients, who are confined to their beds or wheel chairs and who are naturally unable to take part in popular races, are made to believe that they are threatened by CVD. This is absolutely wrong. Those patients are not more prone to CVD than anyone else because in them physical activity cannot cause stress to the point of dysstress. Within their physical limitations they have the normal parasympathetic rebound effect.

## Issue of Clinical Trials

I feel compelled to comment on the repeated demands that so-called scientific clinical trials be performed to demonstrate the effect of testosterone treatment, one group being treated and another not being treated. *Everybody is interested in clinical trials.* Nevertheless, as I will show, it could be harmful if these trials are based upon false assumptions; this might lead to testosterone not being used as often as it should in treatment of CVD. As a result, some patients would be the losers, having to suffer disability, mutilation, or loss of life. Considering the continued demand for the normally accepted form of clinical trials gives me the chance to probe into and discuss the many and various aspects of CVD in relation to clinical trials. The reader can therefore expect to be continuously confronted with these discussions.

Twenty-five years of experience in treating tens of thousands of patients has taught me how careful one must be when assessing the value of testosterone treatment. Our knowledge of circulation is not sufficient to be able to assess an individual's true circulatory condition. There have been countless examples of contradictory approaches to CVD therapy. A vast number of factors are considered to contribute to the development of this so-called disease. Too much cholesterol or too many saturated fats in the diet, too much carbohydrate in the diet, lack of exercise, smoking, high blood pressure, alcohol, air pollution, noise, age, obesity – all these factors and various others have been described as risk or causal factors. With so many and widely differing conditions affecting the etiology of CVD, it is not only extremely difficult to consider it a disease, at least in the usual sense, but it is also extremely difficult to conduct statistically controlled trials. The scientists with whom I have been in contact and who are seriously involved in discovering the true nature of circulatory disease have accepted my approach to this problem. As illustrated by the lines in Fig. 1, we cannot cure CVD as one can other illnesses; we can only improve the condition of a circulatory system which has deteriorated more than usual for a particular age.

Raab (1972 a) elaborated on this confusion.

Regardless of the variously reported nonexistance of thrombi and vascular occlusion in up to more than 50% of myocardial so-called infarctions, and regardless of frequent gross discrepancies between the incidence, degree and location of coronary vascular vs. myocardial structural lesions, such terms as "coronary occlusion," "coronary thrombosis," "coronary atherosclerosis," "coronary heart diesease," "coronary artery disease" or plainly a "coronary" are indiscriminately and interchangeably used in clinical practice and *textbooks* and, especially, in *epidemiologic reports.* Unfortunately, some of the latter, in referring to nonautopsied patient material, glibly employ the terms "atherosclerotic heart disease" or "occlusive coronary disease" or "atherosclerosis," *without any clear proof of the presence or absence of arterial occlusion, or of the degree and actual pathogenic involvement and significance of existing coronary lesions in the individual instances for statistical evaluation.*[1] *A*

---

1 Since Raab's statement of over a decade ago, many similar statements have been made, demonstrating that I am not alone in my criticsm of statistical evaluations.

*dominant element in causation of hypoxia-producing and, consequently, electrolyte-deranging discrepancies between local oxygen supply and consumption consists in the uneconomical, often excessive augmentations of myocardial oxygen consumption that result from the action of adrenosympathetic catecholamines.*
*Profound, potentially pathogenic, and mutally aggravating influences of sympathoadrenal catecholamines and of adrenal corticoids upon the oxygen economy and electrolyte balance of the heart muscle have been intensively investigated over many years. They will be considered specific targets for preventive action against so-called CHD.* This popular, but somewhat worn-out cliché for "coronary heart disease" may more appropriately be read as meaning "cardiac hypoxic dysionism," in keeping with present-day knowledge and concepts.

In a different paper Raab (1949) delivered direct proof that catecholamines lead to hypoxia. For instance, it is common to find angina pectoris attacks in patients with adrenal medullary tumors. These attacks disappear when the tumors are removed surgically. Furthermore, changes in the ECG similar to those seen during angina pectoris attacks can be provoked by injection of adrenaline (epinephrine). The involvement of the autonomic nervous system in the problem of CVD, as described by Raab, makes it much more difficult to conduct clinical trials which can be statistically evaluated.

## Difficulty of Distinguishing CVD from Ageing

If my approach to CVD is accepted, then consideration must be given to the fact that circulatory disease is, in itself, a progressive condition which can be slowed by testosterone together with physical activity. Manifest circulatory disease is interwoven with, and progresses alongside, the deterioration in circulation accompanying ageing. One could imagine that these inseparable processes should make it impossible to prove whether the results of treatment are positive or not by employing the usual medicoscientific methods. If a group of patients receiving treatment is compared with an untreated group, the first may initially show improvement during treatment, but at some later stage they too will show signs of deterioration because the ageing process will overtake both groups, just as it does the rest of humanity. This emphasizes why the two processes cannot be separated and should be a further argument against accepting CVD as a disease similar to other diseases. Treating these patients as I have done over a period of years, I have been able to see that their circulation deteriorates markedly as they grow older, in spite of treatment. However, they kindly remind me of their unhappy state when they came to me many years previously, threatened by amputation which fortunately was made unnecessary by testosterone treatment. Many factors contraindicate comparisons between two groups of subjects. There is nothing as individual as circulation, and consequently it is obvious that each patient *must* act as his own control.

I would like to recount some of the investigations which I carried out. Besides my practice, I have taken an interest in providing physical training to retirees. I found that all these individuals showed signs of impaired circulation, so I decided to compare two groups in their mid-sixties. I took one group about to start physical training and group of patients about to start treatment with testosterone; I was not surprised to observe that the results of my laboratory tests showed virtually no difference between the two groups. For instance, both groups showed similar degrees of impairment of carbohydrate metabolism and ECG abnormalities. The reason *might* have been that my patients who were about to receive testosterone treatment were still leading active lives but had experienced pain, for instance in the form of claudication or angina pectoris, for which they had sought treatment. The members of the other group, having retired, were able to take life more easily, conscious or unconscious of the fact that they were unable to perform the same physical tasks as previously. They had probably accepted this situation, thereby avoiding the symptoms experienced by the active members of the first group, and consequently did not consider themselves to be suffering from CVD; neither did their own doctors.

**Ethical Issues**

Dividing these patients into two groups, the members of the one receiving anabolic steroids, those in the other placebos, would have lead to serious doubt as to the validity of the method. It is well known that placebos may have a positive influence via the autonomic nervous system, which is precisely the system which governs circulation. Consequently the results would have been unreliable. Of course, there is also an ethical reason for not undertaking a two-group trial. How could a physician accept the sight of patients suffering from gangrene and receiving physiological saline instead of testosterone, when we know that the result might be amputation which could have been avoided, in many cases, by testosterone therapy?

Let us try to approach this as a personal problem. If I, for example, should be unfortunate enough to develop gangrene, knowing as we do how testosterone treatment in many cases affects gangrene, I would never permit amputation of my leg instead of testosterone therapy. This is my personal standpoint and a principle which I feel must be applied for the benefit of my patients.

An article written in a medical journal by a well-known scientist comes to mind here. He wrote that if he himself should suffer from some disease which could be succesfully treated with a particular preparation, he would not hesitate to use it on himself and hope to be among those who (according to the trial) were helped by it, even though the effect of this preparation had not been proved statistically significant. He would not "give a damn for the statistics which, in this situation, would appear perfectly ridiculous to him."

Ganong, like many other authors, reports in his *Review of Medical Physiology* (1975, p. 251): "The biological effects of insulin are so far-reaching and complex that they are best illustrated by a consideration of consequences of insulin deficiency." I interpret this to mean that nobody in their right mind would dream of dividing diabetic patients into two groups, treating one with insulin and letting the other group perish, simply because insulin action and the pathogenesis of diabetes mellitus are not fully understood.

I have received many serious offers of cooperation from several universities, where experienced colleagues are now able to appreciate the enormous value of hormone treatment of CVD, which they are willing to support in every possible way. Here they have found a solution which has not been reached by any other means, in spite of enormous economic and scientific efforts. But even though scientists of repute in the USA and elsewhere have expressed admiration for the results of testosterone treatment on CVD, which they have personally witnessed, and although they have shown a positive attitude toward references from medical literature which demonstrate scientifically the favorable effects of testosterone on CVD, nevertheless some of them continue to insist on this division into two groups to *see* how or whether testosterone works. A layman might ask, is not this exactly what they have *seen* with their own eyes? I am constantly being asked, both verbally and in writing, for specifications of dosage and frequency of administration. If I had the opportunity of sitting at ease in quiet conversation with these colleagues, I could make it clear to them what has been going on in my clinic for the past 25 years and make them appreciate the *extremely difficult situation they put me in by asking for clinical trials, dosage, and duration of administration.*

## Difficulty of Evaluating Treatment

A practice with circulatory patients consists of a very varied collection of cases. I would like to mention a few examples starting with a description of a claudication patients, who may be helped by hormones quickly and may not feel the need for further treatment. This case is in the category of *short-term* treatment, but I know from experience that such a patient will probably return for treatment sooner or later because the symptoms have recurred.

There is also the claudication patient who is able to very clearly visualize the terrible results that this apparently harmless condition can lead to. His conception of gangrene is entirely different from that of cardiac infarction, although they are two manifestations of the same disease. Because infarction is invisible to the patient and there are good chances of remission, he does not see it in the same light as gangrene, an infected sore which makes a dramatic impression on everyone who sees it. He may have met acquaintances who have been in hospital with infarction and are now active again, making a bagatelle of their condition and leading a normal life again. In contrast, he knows that a patient with gangrene constantly suffers hideous pain and eventually has to lose a limb, becoming disabled and dependent on others. Should this patient reach that stage, the treatment demanded will be *long term* and both patient and doctor will need great patience (see Figs. 7 and 8). Who would dare to demand of me that I should treat such patients with saline instead of with hormones?

Elsewhere in this book I have mentioned that healed gangrene is only an improved localized symptom of generally poor circulation. In many cases a patient whose gangrene has healed may feel that his health is so much better that he does not return to the clinic for follow-up, but it comes as no suprise to me when his relatives inform me that his life came to an abrupt end because of an infarction that had been indicated on the ECG. It might have been necessary to continue his treatment at a lower dosage. In my opinion this patient cannot be classified together with those who have terminated their treatment but continued medication over a longer period with a lower individual dosage.

A quite different case is the female patient (described on p. 37) whose dosage must continually be adjusted according to her immediate condition. Any suggestion that this type of patient should be excluded from a trial would mean that patients would be selected and not picked at random; therefore the trial would be worthless. All types of patients must, of course, be included.

A middle-aged diabetic female consulted me for gangrene in 1979. The gangrene healed and the patient considered herself cured. This process repeated itself four times during the next 4 years. In such a situation where the patient considers herself cured, can the doctor question this and compel continuation of treatment? (Recently this patient died during an operation for some other condition.) Which category would this patient be classed in at the end of a trial?

# Clinical Findings

The two-group method of testing the value of a preparation has often been criticized, and cytological investigations have been encouraged instead, since they are of paramount importance to physiologists and pathologists and hence to practical medicine [see, for instance, the foreword to Keele and Neil (1961)]. With modern textbooks, students can often more easily understand the nature of CVD than their indoctrinated seniors who cannot, or rather will not, attempt to understand the newer developments in the field of CVD for reasons of prestige. What we are really investigating are the processes of life itself. As I said before, one cannot expect to find the philosopher's stone that will ensure eternal life. It is sufficient to show that medical literature dealing with the effect of testosterone treatment on impaired circulation *supports* this treatment. It is only common sense that emphasis should, above all, be placed on the following objective clinical findings after testosterone therapy:

1. Complete healing of gangrene of the upper and lower extremities, "apparently" an ultimate stage of CVD, occurs in the majority of cases.
2. Improvement of the impaired carbohydrate metabolism has been confirmed by laboratory tests. This impairment is a primary factor in CVD due to overproduction of catecholamines, according to the literature.
3. Milder and fewer attacks of angina pectoris, in many cases, disappear eventually. Cardiac infarction and signs of a lack of oxygen on the ECG tend to be normalized.

Scientific support of these clinical findings is found in many studies. To single out a few, Fliegel (1962) has treated 2,546 CVD patients aged 40–70 with anabolic steroids and found improvement in 75% of the cases (for instance, a decrease in ECG abnormalities). Kalliomäki and Seppälä (1963) have confirmed these results: "22 cardiosclerotic patients have been treated with norandrostenolone decanoate during periods of 1–5 months. In 12 cases a decrease of electrocardiographic abnormalities was observed, in 2 cases these abnormalities increased during the treatment and in 8 cases no change in the electrocardiographic findings was seen during the administration of this anabolic steroid." Similar findings were reported by Hammer (1966), Kutschera-Aichbergern (1966), and Bubenheim (1953). A more randomized double-blind study carried out by Jaffe (1977) also showed a highly significant decrease in ST-segment depression in men treated with testosterone cypionate.

In the treatment of patients with gangrene, one must remember that this is a serious clinical stage of CVD in the extremeties. It must be assumed that fewer positive results can be expected with these patients at stage 3 than with those patients at stages 1 and 2. I presume that any trial should be based on cases where the disease has reached the same stage of development. But what is the criterion for stage 3 patients as to the seriousness of their condition? Should the size of the gangrenous area be measured in square centimeters? The size of a gangrenous area is, however, no indication of the patient's condition since CVD is not confined to the region of the gangrene. CVD affects the entire circulatory system and can become manifest anywhere in the organism. In this very serious pathological stage of the circulatory condition, one cannot exclude the possibility that the patient will die from a heart attack. This often happens and confirms that we are dealing not only with a gangrenous extremity, but with the entire circulation. Consequently, it is clear that the circulation was at a critical stage quite apart form the gangrene. After all, it must be obvious that it is the state of CVD as a whole that we are trying to elucidate.

I have had patients with gangrenous areas the size of peas which have proved to be refractory to treatment, and I have had patients where half the foot has been gangrenous but who have nevertheless been saved from amputation. Another example of the difficulty of assessing the effect of testosterone on pathological circulation is that at the same time we must consider the amount of physical activity undertaken by the patient.

Asking how long treatment of claudication patients must continue reminds me of one of my cases. As mentioned previously, I have run a clinic and treated thousands of patients over the last 25 years, and it is natural that with *so many patients* over *so many years* both doctor and patients must experience moments of doubt. For instance, there was the case of a 55-year-old man whom I had been treating for 3–4 years. I realized that this claudication patient had apparently not benefitted from his long-term testosterone treatment. So I asked him whether he wished to continue, where upon I was given the answer that he insisted on continuing, even though his walking distance had not improved. He told me that he knew several of my patients for whom the hospital had recommended amputation and who had been saved from this step by testosterone treatment. Furthermore, there were members of his family who had been disabled by amputation, so he wished to continue the treatment and was quite satisfied with the result. At least he still had both of his legs. This ordinary workman wrote a chapter on medicine for me, after which I was able to draw my diagram with the two sloping lines; although 4–5 years older biologically than his own age group, his rate of physical deterioration had become normal for ageing again. After 3–4 years of treatment he had returned from a point on line b in Fig. I to the rate of deterioration given by line a. In a two-group trial this patient would have been wrongly included in the category of patients for whom treatment had been ineffective.

Claudication is described as stage 1 of CVD. Many hospitals send their patients home, telling them to wait until the pain becomes unbearable (stage 2) or until gangrene (stage 3) sets in, after which it will be necessary to operate as amputation will then be the only treatment and the only solution. My experience has taught me that this method of procedure must be prevented at all costs and that testosterone treatment ought to be used before amputation regardless of clinical trials.

Previously I discussed a division of individuals at the same age into two groups, one of patients about to receive treatment and the other of retirees about to start physical training. This experiment showed very clearly that there was no definite division between patient and nonpatient, disease or no disease. Yet this is not the case if one goes further down the steeply sloping line b in Fig. 1. Patients become increasingly less able to be physically active and thus cannot stimulate their own testosterone production. When we reach the lowest level, the stage of gangrene, physical activity becomes more or less impossible. Thus the positive results of physical training must decrease in relation to the descent of the line. The mobility of patients is of utmost importance because physical activity is part of the treatment, with or without hormones. This factor is impossible to evaluate in clinical trials.

I tell my claudication patients to exercise as much as possible all the time in order to help the hormones work, but they must not exercise if it is painful because this would cause hypoxia and cellular damage. Anyone who has worked with patients of any age who are confined to bed knows that their muscles atrophy during this period due to a lack of physical exercise. Movement is necessary for the endogenous production of anabolic steroids. This endogenous production decreases due to inactivity as far as gangrenous patients are concerned. Exogenous testosterone is more effective if the patient can move about, and inactivity greatly reduces the possibility of successful testosterone treatment in extreme cases. We must be content to see fewer positive results at stage 3. In such cases a higher dosage of testosterone is justified.

To give examples of treatment with higher dosages, I ask the reader to pay particular attention to two of the cases illustrated in the photographic series. These cases (see Figs. 7 and 8) are similar to many others observed over the years. One of these patients received testosterone treatment for about 3 years, the other for 4. First the pain disappeared, which gave the patients hope so that they continued with the treatment. Today they are able to lead normal lives, eat and sleep naturally, and are happy to have the use of their limbs.

Despite of the good results, we must always remember that what we are fighting against is the continually deteriorating activity of the life processes. The doctor must realize that he must accept defeat where the debility of a patient is stronger than the effect of treatment.

I have mentioned above that endogenous production of testosterone depends on the amount of physical activity. Therefore, two-group trials carried out where one group receives testosterone and the other physical training can only give unrealiable results. Readers who have studied my theories, which are based on my experience and supported by reputed scientists, will appreciate that I find it difficult to understand why physicians working in this field are not acquainted with the extensive literature which emphasizes the fact that physical activity has an effect similar to the administration of testosterone. Therefore this similaritiy *must* blur the results of the two different treatments.


## Individual Nature of Treatment

In the following discussion I will comment in more detail on the relationship between the patient and testosterone treatment. My reflections may have some relevance to controlled clinical trials. The trials which have been carried out included only a small number of patients over a very short period of time; moreover, important factors were not taken into consideration, which resulted in a blurring of the results. These trials were not impressive and were soon forgotten, although the results were more or less positive.

The usual dosage of testosterone for both men and women is mentioned in connection with the photographs (see "Case Studies" and the Appendix), but the maximal dosage can be considerably larger. Naturally it is up to each individual colleague, using normal medical discretion and responsibility, to decide the size of the doses he will use in order to obtain, for instance, the healing of serious gangrene. The rule that the amount depends on the individual case applies to the use of testosterone as well as of insulin. I recall a 50-year-old man for whom I had prescribed 100 mg testosterone suppositories instead of injections. He did not return to my clinic for control, but by chance I met him several months later. In the meantime he had obtained his own supply of the medicine and dosed himself with testosterone ad libitum, that is to say, in doses up to 1 g daily, with the result that his large and serious area of gangrene had healed completely. I never hesitate to give high doses in cases where the gangrene does not heal with smaller amounts.

A skilled and intelligent scientist specializing in CVD recently visited my clinic in Copenhagen and, like others before him who had seen my patients and their prognosis from a hospital, realized that there was a medical alternative to surgery. However, he felt it was necessary to have clinical trials in order for the medical profession as a whole to accept this therapy. He was apparently unswayed by the fact that sufficient scientific evidence to support the use of this preparation has been obtained in the laboratory by studying its corrective action on the metabolic hypoxia which contributes to cardiovascular disturbances. He did, however, agree with me and with the late Sir Hans Krebs that a doctor uses many preparations which have little scientific basis, such as analgesics, sedatives, and tranquilisers, which are prescribed in huge quantities and which can have fatal side effects. He urged me nevertheless to accept clinical trials, which I repeat can be extremely difficult to carry out. When I asked him whether he would recommend a disabling operation (which often rapidly results in death) for his own father rather than testosterone therapy, simply because clinicals trials have not been carried out, he replied that he would try testosterone therapy first of course.

Clinical trials are said to be necessary in order to prove whether testosterone can improve the walking distance of handicapped subjects. Prominent physicians at various universities insist that these trials be carried out over a *very* long period of time and include a *very* large number of patients. According to the Multiple Risk Factor Intervention Trial (MRFIT), these trials should last for *more* than 6–7 years and use *more* than the 12,000 patients of the MRFIT (Multiple Risk Factor Intervention Trial Research Group 1982).

My arguments against these trials are based entirely on my clinical experience and cannot be dismissed without showing a lack of understanding of the CVD problem. It is also experience which tells me that although certain patients will show some improvement in walking distance after 1 year, others will die from myocardial infarction before the trials finish. Improved walking distance, it would appear, is not necessarily the same as improved circulation. On the other hand, the circulatory deterioration with ageing, with the resulting shortened walking distance, will also show itself by the end of a 6–7-year period. I see this daily, with hundreds of patients. When assessing the results of such an investigation, patients with unchanged or shortened walking distances, *although still alive,* would be classed as showing negative results. However, walking distance is not a disease. The aim of such an investigation should be greater insight into circulatory function. These patients live longer, in fact, with their shortened walking distance (but with comparatively better circulation) than those with longer walking distances who die before trials are finished.

It is a pleasure for me as a doctor when my patients are able to lead a relatively normal life in spite of their CVD, although they may be limited by an increasingly shorter walking distance. This is more or less what we must all learn to live with as we grow older. These patients at least avoid the amputation advised in some hospitals. Earlier I argued that the idea that life could be lengthened by physical training is preposterous. How could one actually estimate, before a man started physical training, how long he could be expected to live, and again estimate his expected lifespan after a period of training? *The same applies to the evaluation of circulation. We have, in fact, no standard for comparison since the development of each individual with regard to life, longevity, and circulation is unique.*

## Doctor-Patient Relationship

When I read medical literature concerning CVD I sometimes doubt how much experience the authors of some of these articles have had with CVD patients. This leads me to tell of my own experience with patients. It is true that I take great heart from patients who express their gratitude for the way in which testosterone has helped them. However, it is difficult to say whether my reluctance to share their enthusiasm is unconscious or not. Probably it is because *I* know that I am fighting against superior odds. Sooner or later the patient also will accept the fact that everyone's circulation deteriorates as they grow older. Most patients, as well as the general public, accept this fact. It is amazing that those who have suggested running clinical trials over a period of 6–10 years are not aware of what any layman knows, namely that circulation deteriorates individually with age, a fact which invalidates all such prolonged trials.

About 5 years ago a certain patient first came to consult me. She was about 45 years old, with all the symptoms of poor circulation: ST depression, paresthesia, and cold extremities which kept her awake at night. This female patient presented, as many women do, a lack of pigment and was sensitive to sunlight. This is a typical case, and the patient was soon helped by testosterone therapy. She declared herself not only free of symptoms but also to feel better than before; she was also able to enjoy her sex life again. I was informed that her husband and children felt that she was a happier and healthier person. She started with relatively small doses of testosterone, but on her follow-up visits we discovered that the dosage had to be increased in order to prevent recurrence of the symptoms. As time passed she realized that her general condition was not as good as it had been at the end of the first period of treatment, even though the dosage was higher (with very few side effects). This patient became very depressed again, out of a fear of surgery, as she had been prior to her first visit. This case illustrates the relationship between patient and the doctor who must change the dosage according to the patient's condition; the latter may vary so much that it would be difficult to fit the patient in a clinical trial.

It is as if these patients in some way contact one another and learn how serious this disease can become. When faced with a patient like this, I realize how far we still have to go in the medical profession, and find it difficult to know what to say. In some way I feel guilty. It would be too easy to tell this unhappy soul that she must just learn to live with her illness when in reality I mean that she must learn to die from her illness. Realizing that every possibility of helping has been exhausted makes me feel helpless and frustrated. I feel I have betrayed her confidence. Nevertheless, one has to carry on, trying to help where it is possible but realizing that the illness will always demand its victims. All those who work with a serious disease of this kind understand this feeling.

Most of the patients who come for treatment are well on in age, and most have asked to be discharged from a hospital in order to receive medical treatment from me. These are the most advanced and hopeless cases and yet I am, nevertheless often able to save them from amputation. It is therefore understandable that in *my* position I feel indignant at the demands that clinical trials be conducted before I can try to help these people. Those who favor clinical trials should remember all the arrogant research papers which have stated one thing one day and the opposite the next. I wholeheartedly agree with the statement of the President of The British Cardiac Society, Professor M. F. Oliver (1983), who in his article entitled "Should We Not Forget About Mass Control of Coronary Risk Factors" seems to share my opinion of many so-called scientists, i.e., that they have little knowledge of the *biology and natural history of CVD*. Professor Oliver also remarked: "This does not deter them, whether for commercial or personal reasons, from preaching a calvanistic life-style for us all."

In this discussion of clinical trials, I hope that I have not led my readers to believe that I am against statistics and mathematics in principle. On the contrary, I am very interested in and involved with them. However, I believe that statistics for the sake of statistics, without a thorough understanding of the problem involved, is mere nonsense. Several expert Scandinavian statisticians have stated that it is extremely difficult to establish accurate statistics about CVD because we are dealing with so many unknown factors.

Some final comments may perhaps help to clarify my concept of and opposition to clinical trials made under false assumptions. The kind of statistical evidence that can be used to evaluate testosterone treatment must refer to each individual patient's response and therefore cannot be based on group studies. For this purpose I will describe two patients, both in their mid-fifties, treated for intermittent claudication with hormones. These two women, Ms. X and Ms. Y, both happened to have a walking distance of 200 m. X is in fact a relaxed type of person, who always takes things easy and whose gait is therefore unhurried, while Y is the active type with quick movements and a fast gait. The result of treatment was positive for both women as far as their individual problems were concerned. In other words, the walking distance of both improved considerably, but this would be impossible to demonstrate if the test required that both walk at the same tempo. The two patients have known each other for many years, and Y remarked spontaneously that she has always unconsciously reduced her speed when accompanying

X. No form of treatment can alter the genetically determined circulation; *each CVD patient will always be his own reference.* There is no standard for comparison since the development of each individual's circulation is unique.

I would like to digress here to deal with the widespread assertion that it is impossible to prove how physical training improves the circulation. I believe that I have done this in this book. Such improvement is exactly what athletes attempt to do. They physically train their circulation in order to achieve greater capacity. Here again, capacity is to some degree genetically determined and this is one factor determining competitive capability. With physical training, athletes can reach a limit which cannot be surpassed. Both the X and the Y types of athletes have their own individual maximums which they cannot exceed. These maximums can only be compared with each individual's own previous and present performances. *Again, each person is his own reference.* Even an active athlete progresses, of course, down line a in Fig. 1 and must give way to a younger athlete sonner or later. The use of hormones to increase athletes' physical capacity in the world of sports is well known.

Returning to the X- and Y-type females, I do not confine myself to what patients, in this instance the two women, tell me about the subjective effects of the treatment. Clinical trials are conducted daily in my clinic. The treatment I give helps in almost all cases of ordinary claudication. There is nothing exceptional about this since the results are in accordance with physiology. I ascertain whether patients attending for follow-up have increased their walking distances, whether their ECG abnormalities have more or less disappeared, whether their glucose tolerance has improved, and whether other negative symptoms have improved. I also test whether decreased enzyme activity affecting carbohydrate metabolism has been increased by hormone therapy. This is, in my opinion, the correct scientific way of carrying out clinical trials.

It would be extremely difficult to persuade me as a member of the medical profession to take a group of 20 patients suffering, for instance, from gangrene and claudication, and divide them into two groups, treating the people in one group in order to compare it with the other, untreated group. I do not wish to treat my patients and fellow human beings as if they were rats. Actually this is illegal. When a patient visits his doctor he does so because his health has become so bad that he is in need of immediate help and believes, rightly, that he will receive the treatment to which he is entitled. Once again, based on 25 years experience, I can say that the condition of people with circulatory disease who are forced to consult their doctor because of some localized symptom is so poor that the disease can manifest itself at any time in – in addition to claudication or gangrene – a myocardial infarction which constantly threatens them, as indicated by ECG abnormalities. There are examples of follow-up appointments which have not been kept because death due to cardiac infarction or cerebral hemorrhage had overtaken the patient. However, should a patient on physiological saline die from cardiac infarction or cerebral hemorrhage during clinical trials, I do not believe I could continue to serve as a doctor, having refrained from correctly treating the patient with hormones. I would consider myself to some extent guilty of his death. Or imagine that a gangrene patient is given salt water instead of medical treatment which is known to have helped thousands of patients. If an amputation does not

prove fatal, he will be disabled for the rest of his life. This terrible fate could have been avoided. What would such a patient think and feel about doctors who have allowed this disastrous situation to remain untreated and to have ruined his life?
After having described these and many other examples of circulatory cases receiving varying dosages of testosterone to colleagues demanding clinical trials and details on dosage and the duration of treatment, I then ask them: "Would it not be far better for you to take it upon yourself to treat your own CVD patients with hormones, in order to acquire the necessary personal experience with patients' reactions. *Then* you could decide how or whether you could carry out double blind trials with these unfortunate people."
It is reasonable to assume that if my positive results inspire a reexamination of my treatment using testosterone, this should be carried out on my terms, that is to say, in the same way that I treat my patients and not in a haphazard manner. I have achieved these good results by treating my patients individually. To me it is not clinical trials but the *patients that comes first*.

## Lack of Pigment

Several specific observations concerning testosterone and estrogen deserve special attention. Among my patients I have found that those suffering from prostate cancer, and therefore receiving treatment with estrogen, show signs of eunuchism with a tendency to fatness, development of mammae, change of voice, and an apparent lack of pigment giving them a pale complexion. Incidentally, eunuchs are prone to CVD. In this connection, therefore, it is interesting to mention that in my clinic female patients who tan poorly and get sunburned easily need a higher dosage of testosterone to obtain a positive result. As a rule these female patients have very few side effects, even when treated with high doses of testosterone.
Remarkably, this fascinating issue was discussed as long ago as 1938–1939. Hamilton and co-workers published two articles on testosterone and tanning (Hamilton and Hubert 1938; Edwards et al. 1939). This is a field where future research may reveal more about the effects of testosterone. In the article from 1938, the authors mentioned a study of three surgically castrated and four hypogonadal men.

Before treatment the skin in all but two cases was of a characteristic pasty, sallow color, gray and lacking in pink tinge. This was most pronounced in the castrated men. After treatment with testosterone propionate there was a rapid flushing, followed by increased oiliness of the skin and growth of hair on the face, chest, abdomen, arms and legs. All patients presented a more tanned appearance, particularly of the face, neck, hands and exposed parts of the skin. Part of this increased pigmentation is due to "developing" of pigment from previous exposure... From studies of men with low amounts of testicular secretion it appears that male hormone substance exerts a "developing" action upon the rather colorless material which is laid down in the skin following exposure to the sun or sun-lamp. This "developing" action may be exerted as late as five months after exposure. This indicates that tanning may be a "photographic-like process" of "exposure" and "development," with the sex hormone acting to "develop" color-lacking material laid down in the skin by exposure. Further, the pigmentation is not established continuously but will fade upon cessation of hormone treatment and reappear upon later resumption of treatment.

I have made similar observations with many of my patients. They tell me jokingly that they can even get a tan by candlelight.

To quote the second article (Edwards et al. 1939):

In as serious a condition as vascular insufficiency of the extremities, any procedure which gives promise of being effective in treatment deserves early trial of its usefulness. In spite, therefore, of the small number of cases of arterial disease that we have treated with testosterone propionate, we feel justified in making this preliminary report. Our attention was directed to the general vascular effect of testosterone propionate while studying the skin changes in human male castrates... We have now treated 7 male patients having organic vascular disease with crystalline testosterone propionate... Each of these patients with vascular disease showed a lack of skin arterialization by spectrophotometry which involved not only the diseased limbs but also the entire body. The administration of testosterone propionate produced a marked change. As in the case of castrates, the spectrophotometric curves after treatment showed in early and decided arterialization of the cutaneous blood. Moreover, the after-treatment curves like-wise showed an inconstant diminution in the volume of blood in the more venous areas of the body. Other objective evidence of favorable changes was an increase in the systolic pressure of from 6 to 26 mm of mercury in the hypotensive members of this group, and a lowering of hypertensive blood pressures in two cases. The ulceration in 1 patient has healed, the second has greatly improved. There was marked improvement in the walking ability of all the patients, with delay or abolition of intermittent claudication. Two patients were no longer subject to night pain, which had troubled them previously. Subjectively, the patients reported an increased activity and a feeling of optimism, results similar to those reported previously with male-hormone treatment.

# Other Findings

## So-called Biochemical Risk Factors

Elevated levels of biochemical substances such as cholesterol and triglycerides, along with decreased fibrinolytic activity, are often associated with CVD and are thus referred to as risk factors. This does not necessarily mean that they cause CVD. They may well be secondary changes only providing indications of a more basic underlying metabolic imbalance; influencing one of them will not automatically improve or cure the clinical disorder any more than turning off a fire alarm will put out the fire. Nevertheless, it is usually encouraging when the levels of these risk factors are reduced in the course of testosterone therapy. This was observed nearly 20 years ago with testosterone when the steroid consistently reduced serum cholesterol (Møller 1977) and increased blood fibrinolytic activity. Without going into details, is has been proven that the daily content of cholesterol in the diet has no appreciable effect on plasma cholesterol levels.
This relationship was summarized at a WHO symposium in Madrid in 1972.

A number of compounds are available which, when administered orally, will raise and sustain the level of fibrinolytic activity significantly. Most successful in this regard are the anabolic steroids and the oral hypoglycemic agents. Ethylestrenol and phenoformin are the most active among the two groups and when used in combination they induce enhanced levels of fibrinolytic activity (approximately five times normal) which can be maintained for periods of several years without any evidence of the untoward consequences of excessive fibrinolysis. This combination also produces a reduction of plasma fibrinogen of approximately 25%, a decrease in platelet adhesiveness, and a significant fall in serum cholesterol. To date there has been little interest in extending or exploiting these findings or in evaluating this form of prophylactic therapy. Most of current endeavours focus upon the evaluation of agents capable of inhibiting platelet function since most coronary thrombi are believed to be platelet initiated. This lack of enthusiasm for undertaking large-scale clinical trials to evaluate prophylactic fibrinolytic therapy is influenced by uncertainty about the beneficial effects of available fibrinolytic agents and lack of knowledge of their mechanism of action.

Elevated levels of plasma fibrinogen are now one of the most widely used risk factors in coronary heart disease according to Meade and Chakrabarti (see Mead et al. 1979), who have published several reports that they have used testosterone to obtain improved fibrinolysis.
Davidson et al. (1972) have suggested that it is unnecessary to combine steroid with phenformin, especially as the former has fibrinolytic action of its own. At the EOCCD we have also proved that testosterone is the substance having the primary effect on fibrinolysis (Winther 1965). The same author (Winther 1966) reported in another article: "I report here a study to determine whether repeated physical training can induce sustained activation of blood fibrinolysis. In all persons except one, there was a clear shortening of the lysis time during each exercise

session, but there was no sustained effect." Here is another example that testosterone and physical activity have similar metabolic effects.

I want to emphasize that the parameters of CVD, such as those mentioned previously, are *interrelated and interdependent*. There is no sense in affecting just one of the parameters, for instance, cholesterol. Tampering with this one factor might have serious consequences. For example, Professor M. F. Oliver (1981) of the Royal Infirmary, Edinburgh, stated in an interview with the Danish newspaper *Berlingske Tidende* that it is not known why the cholesterol level increases on ageing. There may be a correlation to diet or an adaption to the influence of Western life style. Organisms cannot exist without cholesterol, which takes part in all cell functions. If we interfere with this system, e.g., medically, the result may be that we decrease resistance to infection; we may even accelerate the ageing process.

Testosterone, for instance, decreases the cholesterol level and affects all the other parameters positively, e.g., by increasing fibrinolytic activity. It is unnecessary to go into details, but the increased cholesterol level seen in CVD is associated with anaerobic metabolism and can therefore be corrected by testosterone.

In this regard, a study has been reported in which "the concentration of cholesterol in the blood of 300 male patients between the ages of 41–82, with clinically recognizable circulatory diseases", were treated with 250 mg testoviron depot three times weekly. Specifically, it was reported that "in 83% of the circulatory patients cholesterol concentration in the blood fell during androgen treatment to an average of 74% of the concentration before treatment. The fall is apparently independent of the cholesterol level before treatment since no greater fall was observed in 7 patients with very high initial cholesterol values (Møller 1977a, pp. 2, 4). The analytical work in this study was carried out at the hormone laboratory of the State Hospital, Copenhagen.

## Influence of Testosterone on Connective Tissue

I previously mentioned a publication by Sobel and Marmorston (1958) and quoted important paragraphs from it, but postponed discussion of their contribution until now, when my theories have been explained.[1] In that publication the process of ageing is divided into three stages. The third stage is described as the "ageing syndrome – in which the clinical evidence of ageing becomes apparent and antianabolic influences soon predominate." This agrees with my model, depicted in Fig. 1, in which line a indicates the involution of life processes associated with ageing.

According to Sobel and Marmorston, the decrease in hexosamine-collagen (H–C) ratio in connective tissue with advancing age (Fig. 2) leads to an insufficient amount of oxygen passing through the connective tissue and reaching the cells. Again, this is in agreement with my theory that with ageing there is a tendency to anaerobic metabolism, which causes impaired carbohydrate metabolism. This is also indicated by line b in Fig. 1. An oxygen deficiency means a decrease in the synthesis of testosterone from cholesterol, which corresponds to the statement by

---

1 The manuscript for this book was ready to be sent to the publisher when I came across this article, which provides further scientific support for the treatment of CVD with testosterone.

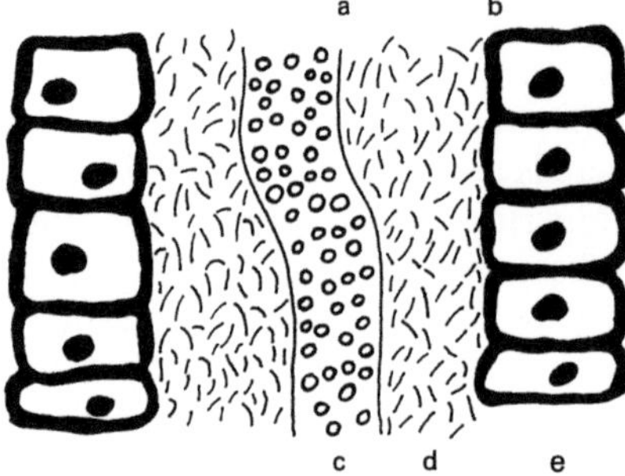



**Fig. 2.** Schematic drawing illustrating the important location of connective tissue (*d*) between the capillaries and parenchymal cells (*e*). *a* Capillary membrane, *b* cell membrane, and *c* blood

Sobel and Marmorston that: "The fact that the excretion of androgens and ketosteroids diminishes with age is well documented by numerous investigators."
I have attached importance to showing that we are dealing with similar qualitative involutions in both lines a and b in Fig. 1 – meaning that line b expresses accelerated involutions. I see here a certain agreement with the comment by Pincus that "aging and certain chronic stress conditions tend to diminish the output of certain urinary steroids. The simple conclusion would be that in aged persons the decrement is the effect of the cumulative stresses of living. In states of chronic stress this effect is telescoped" (quoted in Sobel and Marmorston 1958). Sobel and Marmorston report further that "Pincus and co-workers have pointed out that the excretion of urinary corticoids does not diminish as rapidly with time" as the excretion of androgens and ketosteroids. I interpret this to indicate an increased cortisol concentration which, according to medical textbooks, leads to a decrease in insulin activity, i.e., again to impaired carbohydrate metabolism. Once more my theories are in agreement with Sobel and Marmorston's description; they find an increased corticoid-ketosteroid (Co/K) ratio in patients who have suffered a myocardial infarction (CVD). "Calculation of the ratio of corticoids to ketosteroids... revealed the expected finding that this ratio increased with time [see line a in Fig. 1]. It was considerably elevated in the patients [see line b in Fig. 1." I have demonstrated decreased glucose tolerance in my patients.
It can be seen that the H/C ratio is under the influence of the Co/K ratio from the fact that decreased gonadal activity leads to a negative nitrogen balance and affects "the soluble ground substance which is a part of the metabolic pool." Sobel and Marmorston report further that:

The problem of hormonal control of ground substance polysaccharide appears not to be separate from the problem of hormonal influences on nitrogen metabolism. Changes within the connective tissue may be considered to be permanent with regard to those involving the fibrillar components and potentially reversible with regard to those involving the ground substance.

In other words, androgens increase the H/C ratio and therefore diminish the "susceptibility to atherosclerosis". The same endocrine metabolic processes appear during surgical stress: increased Co/K ratio, impaired carbohydrate metabolism, and negative nitrogen balance. Thus the decrease in the H/C ratio with ageing and in disease depends on anabolic and antianabolic influences.

My concept of CVD illustrated by Fig. 1 may conform to the final comments in

Sobel and Marmorston's article:

These studies have no more than dented the surface of a vast, intricate problem. Perhaps they will one day help us to understand some of the factors which in the ageing process of man cause dissociation of chronological time from biological time and the well-known observation that life experiences play a role in establishing this dissociation. In referring to our definition of ageing, perhaps the slight note of optimism contained therein does not seem unfounded.

I believe that the slight note of optimism was not unfounded as clinical results with testosterone have demonstrated a reduction in the dissociation between chronological age and biological age – in other words, lifted line b up to line a in Fig. 1 and made the author's dream of overcoming this dissociation come true.

*Anticoagulants.* I would like to take this opportunity to describe some of my clinical experiences. At present I am treating a number of patients who have had a thrombus removed from one of the iliac arteries (thrombendarterectomy) in order to "cure" their CVD. Postoperatively their conditions has become aggravated, leaving them only with the prospect of amputation because the operation led to a more widespread occlusion of the arteries in question. I treat these patients with large doses of testosterone, and it is amazing to observe how fast the positive effects set in. I am unable to make a prognosis for these patients, one of the reasons being that the cases often slip out of my hands, treatment being continued elsewhere. The latest patient came from Spain. After only two weeks improvement was evident. I doubt, however, that I will learn anything about the further progress of this particular patient. These patients show a decrease in glucose tolerance prior to treatment which improves strikingly with testosterone treatment, that is, they show a tendency to improved oxygen uptake.

Thrombendarterectomy patients are given anticoagulants, which are claimed to be controlled scientifically using the so-called prothrombine index; the term "anticoagulants" here does not refer to heparin. I worked abroad with anticoagulants in research, and when I started treating CVD patients, anticoagulant treatment was "in." In the meantime it seems to have lost ground because of serious criticism from various parties. I cannot see any scientific basis for this kind of treatment, which simply amounts to interfering with the natural metabolism of the liver. Do the doctors advising this treatment have any idea of the harm it may cause by affecting the enzyme activity of the liver? Anticoagulants may produce very serious or fatal side effects such as gastric, renal, or cerebral hemorrhage.

The best that one can say about anticoagulants is that there should be a prophylactic effect against the formation of thrombi, and this has not yet been proved. Anticoagulants are said to dilute blood, whatever is meant by that. With testosterone one interferes directly with the inert collagen factor; this is thus an active destructive process of the so-called thrombi.

*Fibrinolytic Activity.* An increase in fibrinolytic activity from testosterone is scientifically well documented, both based on work in my own laboratories and on the results of research by other well-known scientists. This kind of treatment is recommended in a WHO report (1972) mentioned in this book. Sobel and Marmorston (1958) have worked with connective tissue and the relation between hexosamine and collagen, the H-C ratio. Testosterone administration leads to an increase in the H-C ratio, which we have seen is of importance for cellular oxygen uptake, i.e., for an improvement of CVD. There is a decrease in the inert collagen fraction, which favors the active hexosamine fraction. Furthermore, testosterone builds up active muscular tissue and in this way prevents necrosis and improves the oxygen supply to the damaged tissue by increasing the H-C ratio. In 1976 Gudbjarnason et al. published an article entitled "Metabolic Changes in Infarcted and Non-Infarcted Myocardium During the Post-Infarction Period," reporting that scar formation in cardiac muscle is markedly reduced in animals treated with anabolic steroids and that collagen formation is reduced by 26%.

# Prophylaxis

Up to now I have discussed how the damage caused by CVD can be repaired once it has become manifest, but it is of course even more important to concentrate on the prevention of damage or, as it is commonly expressed, "How can I avoid a heart attack?" Here I feel very critical of what so-called medical science would have us believe.

I clearly recall how my brilliant professor of medicine at the University of Copenhagen defined a heart attack as the ultimate stage of angina pectoris, and I should like to add that gangrene is the ultimate stage of claudication. Amputation is traditionally given as the only therapeutic solution for gangrene and now bypass operations are becoming widespread in the treatment of angina pectoris. But here again it appears that surgery for medical problems leads to fatal results although those who defend surgery in these cases claim that it gives the patient a chance of survival and of living longer. Yet there is no justification for the assertion that patients' lives have been lengthened. Medical treatment with anabolic steroids has been used in numerous cases with undisputable results to improve patients' lives. I personally have treated thousands of cases where the attacks became milder, less frequent, and eventually disappeared entirely, with the ST depression on the ECG being normalized.

Some of the drawbacks of bypass operations have been pointed out by Atkinson (1983). "Atherosclerosis progresses more rapidly in bypass grafts than it does in native coronary arteries. It may take a person 50 years to build up enough atherosclerotic plaque to clog his coronary arteries, whereas it may take only three or four years to clog his bypass grafts." Atkinson found further that "in 12 cases of bypass operation total occlusion of the graft occurred soon after surgery." The majority of patients died from heart disease. "We don't know if their deaths were related to changes seen in their bypass grafts, or because of atherosclerosis in their native coronary arteries."

In Japan the prophylactic use of testosterone has been suggested for cases where factors indicating the development of CVD have been ascertained in the laboratory. I can accept this if clinical signs such as claudication and angina pectoris are present. Nevertheless, I am reluctant to use testosterone prophylactically until the results of further research inspired by my approach have been achieved.

The environment has a great influence on the development of CVD as well as on the development of many other diseases. Although we ourselves have created the circumstances under which we live, I do not believe that the individual can do a great deal to counteract their influence; major changes in the environment can only be effected by political means.

During the second symposium held by the EOCCD on circulatory disease in 1977, which took place in the House of Lords in London, I made a speech to leading politicians and a selected group of the best scientists from the field of circulatory disease. I finished this speech (Møller 1977 b) by saying:

"As president of the EOCCD I have now set the ball rolling for discussion, and I hope that by the end of this meeting it will be possible to state that we have now got a solid foundation on which to build. I must also involve the politicians in this debate, since the organization consists of both politicians and scientists. It is universally agreed that vascular diseases have become a socioeconomic problem. Man has an established life span with broad individual variations which arise from inherited characteristics that form the process of getting older and the process of dying, and are beyond medical control. Nevertheless, this descending curve of life is accelerated by the modern way of living in our society. As it is accepted that there is a link between these diseases and rapid development of society today, with statistics showing that the situation is steadily getting worse, this is where the politicians can, and must, take action to halt these processes by attempting to alter society, to make it more suitable for a sound and healthy existence. Therefore I will end my causerie by making my most sincere appeal to the politicians. We doctors must admit that, up to now, we have been going from one wrong track to another. We are inclined to think that this problem can be solved on a purely scientific basis, which it cannot. That is why we need the co-operation of you, the politicians. You can see more clearly, with fresh minds and common sense, how to attack – and I quote Mr. Spicer again – this "international enemy.""

But what can people do for themselves? First of all, they should keep themselves in good shape by, for instance, staying physically active. More than 20 years ago I started an institution with facilities for voluntary supervised physical activity, which is still functioning with more than 2,000 visits a week.

Although the subject of diet is complex, I feel that CVD is fundamentally a metabolic rather than a dietary problem. Nevertheless, it is advisable to restrict caloric intake to avoid overweight, and ensure sufficient protein and vegetables in the diet. Gudbjarnasson et al. (1976) found that protein-free diet results in a significant diminution of ATP levels in connection with treatment with anabolic steroids. Above all, people should stop smoking and avoid or reduce alcohol consumption to a minimum, not allowing it to become a daily habit. I do not claim to have the answer or solution for a healthy life, but everyone should use his individual common sense as to how to live in a healthy manner without making life so dull that the cure is worse than the illness.

# Medical Treatment

I have mentioned the unfortunate patients who, with confidence in the medical profession, have been treated surgically with fatal consequences. It is not possible to obtain reliable statistics on the results of vascular surgery. Yet even if the operation in some cases shows an apparent positive effect on a localized CVD "attack," other disastrous results will dominate to such an extent that they make these risky operations unjustifiable. I am well aware of what is said to some of the patients before surgery. The doctors warn the patients of possible risks, but this is absolutely no excuse for their actions. The odds are against the patient, who is not able to judge the medical situation. He has turned to the doctor for professional help, who claims that there is no alternative treatment. Let me emphasize that I am, of course, not accusing any colleague of willfully causing injury to the patient. These colleagues are convinced that they act in the best interest of the patient. In this book I have pointed out an alternative way to help the patient without the risk of irreparable damage. Nonetheless, I have to remind my colleagues that this disease is quite different from those usually met in medical practices. First of all, this treatment requires patience. Sometimes positive results are rapidly achieved, but in a few cases treatment must continue for a very long time; fortunately, these cases are rare. From the color photographs (see the Appendix) you can see that two patients were treated for more than 3 years before the gangrene healed. These are not isolated cases here in my clinic. A unique degree of contact is made between the doctor and such a patient.

There are days when I doubt whether treatment will be successful. Perhaps my expressions disclose this doubt, making the patient, strangely enough, feel that it is now his turn to console me by reminding me of the fact that there has, after all, been improvement in comparison with his condition at the beginning of treatment. He has made up his mind to avoid amputation as long as there is some progress. The fact that the patient is so involved in the treatment that he never feels unhappy over the seriousness of his situation makes the doctor's job easier and thus enables the doctor to share his hope. This is a happy ending to an extremely difficult issue.

This experience reveals the story of a true medical contribution instead of clinical trials and statistics, which cure nothing and may only serve the purpose of discouraging the patients as well as the doctor. I have warned against clinical trials and statistics, and if those who support them later comprehend that these are based on false assumptions they will surely regret the disaster that may have been caused by their unyieldingly adhering to an absolute demand. I feel that clinical trials and statistics have become a complex for certain university people. With regard to treatment, male patients are initially treated with 250 mg testosterone enanthate with depot effect, three times weekly. Female patients are treated similarly but with 100 mg, having willingly accepted the risk of the side effects they had been warned of in advance. Dosage is gradually reduced as the patient's condition improves, or increased if required by the situation.

The many offers to carry out research from, among others, a number of universities in the United States could perhaps be accepted, with the purpose of achieving the same results with female patients, using lower dosages over longer periods and consequently avoiding side effects. From my own experience I know that there is potential for improvement.

Edema caused by fluid and sodium chloride retention may appear, but diuretics counteract this satisfactorily. In such cases of edema, or polycythemia, a short pause in the treatment is required.

In my large practice neither I nor any of the physicians associated with my clinic throughout the years have observed a single case of cancer due to testosterone treatment. All endocrinologists agree that testosterone is not carcinogenic. But what about estrogens? At times it is difficult to understand medical science. Estrogens are sold in high quantities throughout the world and it has been proven that they have a carcinogenic effect. Nevertheless, they are used as a medical preparation where the doctor finds it necessary and suitable. Estrogens increase the high-density lipoprotein level in plasma, a state which should prove favorable for avoiding circulatory disease. However, there have been claims that these substances increase the possibility of CVD. This is confirmed by prostate cancer patients who become prone to circulatory disease when treated with estrogens. Women who have developed circulatory disease as a result of estrogens have sued drug manufacturers, but is it the manufacturers who prescribe the medicine and treat the patients?

# Testosterone and Plasma Lipids

Perhaps the following presentation of the results of my own investigations could alter their attitude and help to persuade them not to be so refractory concerning the immediate importance of clinical trials until the correct conditions for the execution of these trials can be agreed on, if they are to be carried out at all.

It has been suggested that CVD arises from a shift in the normal balance between anabolic and catabolic metabolic processes in favor of the catabolic, and that this shift normally takes place gradually throughout a person's lifetime. An acceleration in the rate of the shift can, however, be counteracted by the administration of substances having an anabolic effect. I, and many others, have pointed out that anabolic testosterone is capable of slowing this acceleration toward a catabolic imbalance and of leading the metabolic processes back to their normal condition, i.e., to the condition corresponding to the age of the patient.

By having referred to numerous scientific publications from recognized university authorities, I have disappeared out of the picture of argumentation. It should nonetheless be obvious that it provides me with great satisfaction to see that those who have worked seriously with the CVD problem have the same concept that I have, namely, that a dominance of catabolic processes results in hypoxia which means anaerobic metabolism. Consequently, insufficient oxaloacetic acid is available for the oxidation of acetyl-coenzyme A (CoA) resulting in an increased plasma lipid concentration; this can be seen with the *naked eye* (see Fig. 3).

With my encouragement, one university in Denmark has engaged in carrying out glucose tolerance tests and another in testing plasma lipid concentrations in patients receiving testosterone therapy. The pathological glucose tolerance has been shown to be strikingly improved by testosterone; this clearly demonstrates a shift from anaerobic to aerobic metabolism, producing sufficient oxaloacetic acid for the oxidation of acetyl-CoA.

In front of me are two excellent physiology textbooks – *Samson Wright's Applied Physiology* (Keele and Neil 1961) and J. H. Green's *An Introduction to Human Physiology* (1976), with diagrams of the Krebs cycle. I feel tempted to describe these diagrams as "silent pictures" which show the two alternative pathways for the dissimilation of fat, the anaerobic which leads to increased plasmalipid concentration and the aerobic which conducts fat into the Krebs cycle of normal metabolism.

We now have photographs of test tubes containing plasma lipids which tell us – like "talking pictures" – what is going on in metabolism. Our attention is attracted by the way in which the creamy white opaque liquid gradually becomes clearer and clearer and eventually transparent; please note that this occurs concurrently with improvement in glucose tolerance. Furthermore, we must stress that these changes appear concurrently with, and because of, testosterone administration. Most important, and more essential than anything else, is the fact that

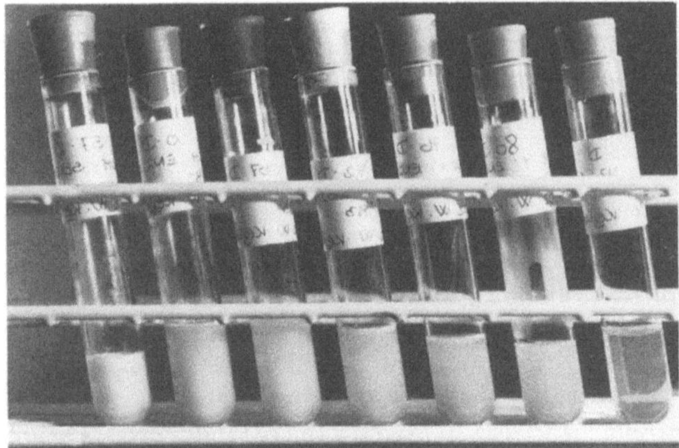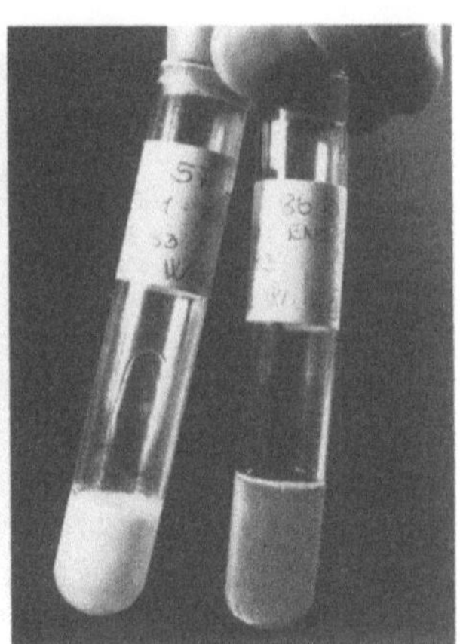

**Fig. 3. a** The gradual clearing illustrates the gradual use of plasma lipids in the accelerated carbohydrate metabolism and the gradual transition from anaerobic to aerobic metabolism caused by testosterone treatment. **b** The plasma before and after treatment

the patient's circulation also improves concurrently. The claudication patient walks without difficulty, angina pectoris attacks slowly disappear, gangrene heals, and signs of hypoxia on the ECG are normalized. The process which we can see going on in the test tubes gives life to the diagrams of the Krebs cycle in the textbooks. Everyone involved in these experiments becomes so fascinated by this demonstration of the CVD problem, superlative in its simplicity, that they get carried away by their enthusiasm. The photographs in Fig. 3 illustrate the process in such a fantastic manner that they border on magic; they demonstrate the chemical processes, distinctly confirming the classical phrase that "the fats only burn in the flame of the carbohydrates."

Up to now a university professor has shown medical students test tubes filled with opaque, creamy plasma but has not been able to give a medical solution for the normalization. I well understand medical students when they so frankly declare that they are bored and fed up with repeatedly being given so many different hypotheses and theories concerning a solution to the CVD problem; this frustration makes them feel that what they are taught changes with fashion, like hats and dresses, as in the quotation from Thomas Jefferson cited in the Preface.

# Parameters of CVD

It is exciting to discover that by going beneath the surface of the CVD problem it is possible to interpret the disease in quite different ways. I feel that it is my duty to inform my patients' regular doctors of my laboratory results and the treatment I have given. The interesting thing is that in several cases I have experienced that a patient has been told by his doctor that, according to my laboratory results, he has been suffering from "diabetes" which the testosterone treatment has cured. In other words, the testosterone normalized the impaired carbohydrate metabolism. These colleagues have explained to patients, furthermore, that the simultaneous disappearance of the circulatory symptoms is natural since they were the result of the "diabetes." It is completely irrelevant to me whether the patient's condition is termed CVD or "diabetes." Does the hen come before the egg or the egg before the hen? Important is that scientific experiments show that testosterone normalizes glucose tolerance.

I have also had patients who attended a medical laboratory of their own initiative in order to have their cholesterol levels checked. I had already done this, but people still suffer from cholesterol neurosis. At the laboratory the same story was repeated. Here the doctor tells the patient encouragingly that his hypercholesterolemia has been normalized by the testosterone treatment and that this is the reason the circulatory symptoms have also disappeared.

I have previously explained that the parameters, or so-called risk factors, are intercorrelated and interdependent; that is to say, if one is affected the others will also be affected making the choice of which one is used to express the disease a matter of preference. Time and time again I have claimed that CVD is not a disease which can be compared with other diseases and that it is a very vague and imprecise term. Dozens of etiologies have been suggested, and I have quoted Raab's (1972a) article about the even greater number of false diagnostic terms. It would perhaps be a good idea if the misleading term "CVD" could be replaced by, for instance, Raab's term "cardiac hypoxic dysionism," which not only describes the disease exactly, but also includes the pathogenesis. Counteraction of hypoxia by testosterone restores aerobic metabolism; testosterone thus provides the decisive basis for this method of therapy.

# Conclusion

Looking at what I have written in this book, I must thank fate for providing me with such a large number of publications, many of the highest quality, which I have been able to call upon to substantiate the anabolic effects of testosterone on metabolism and therefore its positive effect on CVD.

My gratitude is directed first and foremost to my patients, whose clinical results have encouraged my to search deeper into the nature of circulatory disease. I always remind the medical students working with me that it is not the doctor who puts the symptoms together to make a disease. In each individual case it is, in fact, the patient who experiences the disease and is therefore best able to convey to the doctor the problems involved. In this book I have told how a patient helped me to look at CVD not as a disease but rather as a part of the process of life. I cannot emphasize strongly enough the necessity for respect and humility in our relationship to patients, who play the most important and decisive roles in our profession. An understanding attitude toward the patient followed by the appropriate action has priority over epidemiological and clinical trials which have not yet produced any results.

In summarizing my theories and beliefs, I would like to make the following main points:

Testosterone is the life-giving and life-maintaining substance. Scientists studying the evolution of life suggest that a unique role might have been played by cyclopentanoperhydrophenanthrene, the nucleus of which is contained in testosterone. Furthermore, in embryology testosterone has a unique role and is an essential factor in human development (Neumann 1977). The important role of testosterone was well described by Bardin (1979):

> Once the androgen-receptor complex is formed, it is transferred to the nucleus where it binds to specific sites on chromatin. The binding site for the steroid-receptor complex has been termed the nuclear acceptor site. Interaction of the steroid-receptor complex with its receptor results in a striking increase in the nuclear metabolism. This includes an increase in chromatin activity, an increase in the number of initiation sites on chromatin, and an increase in the synthesis of all classes of RNA. These events lead to increased transfer of RNA to cytoplasm which results in protein synthesis, cellular growth, and differentiated function.

This quotation demonstrates a concept which is generally accepted.

Testosterone is essential for the formation of proteins and enzymes, for instance those in the Krebs cycle, which are the fundamental basis for normal metabolism, maximal ATP production, and optimal circulation. It is the basic means of helping CVD patients. Knowing that life processes depend on testosterone and that CVD is a disturbance of the life processes, it can only be logical to concentrate research on this substance. This is especially true since I, and many others, have achieved thousands of convincing positive clinical results in the practice of hormone therapy.

In spite of all other research carried out at enormous expense, it appears that the most effective way at the moment of helping people who suffer from CVD is testosterone treatment. All other methods that have been tried have proved relatively ineffective. In this connection I would like to mention that no one has yet been able to convince me that CVD is a surgical problem. It should not be necessary to have to tell physicians that the problem *is a medical one*.

I would like to conclude by asking: Has the time not come to stop talking about testing testosterone in clinical trials and concentrate instead on biochemical research into the action of testosterone on CVD, the result of which has been demonstrated in this book? In this way, I assure you, we will also obtain sufficient scientific evidence for the use of testosterone in therapy, and this should help to alter the attitude of young physicians and medical students toward CVD.

# Appendix
## Photographic Presentation of Patients with Gangrene

Over the past 25 years, thousands of patients have been successfully treated with testosterone preparations in my clinic in Copenhagen, Denmark. The following photographs depict nine patients with gangrenous ulcers that are representative of the responses of the many patients attending the clinic for treatment of vascular disease. All nine had been discharged from a hospital with amputation recommended as the only solution. All subsequently became free from pain and were able to lead normal lives and participate in suitable occupations.
The photographs of the first three patients (Figs. 4–6) show gradual results; the others (Figs. 7–12) show the condition before and after treatment.

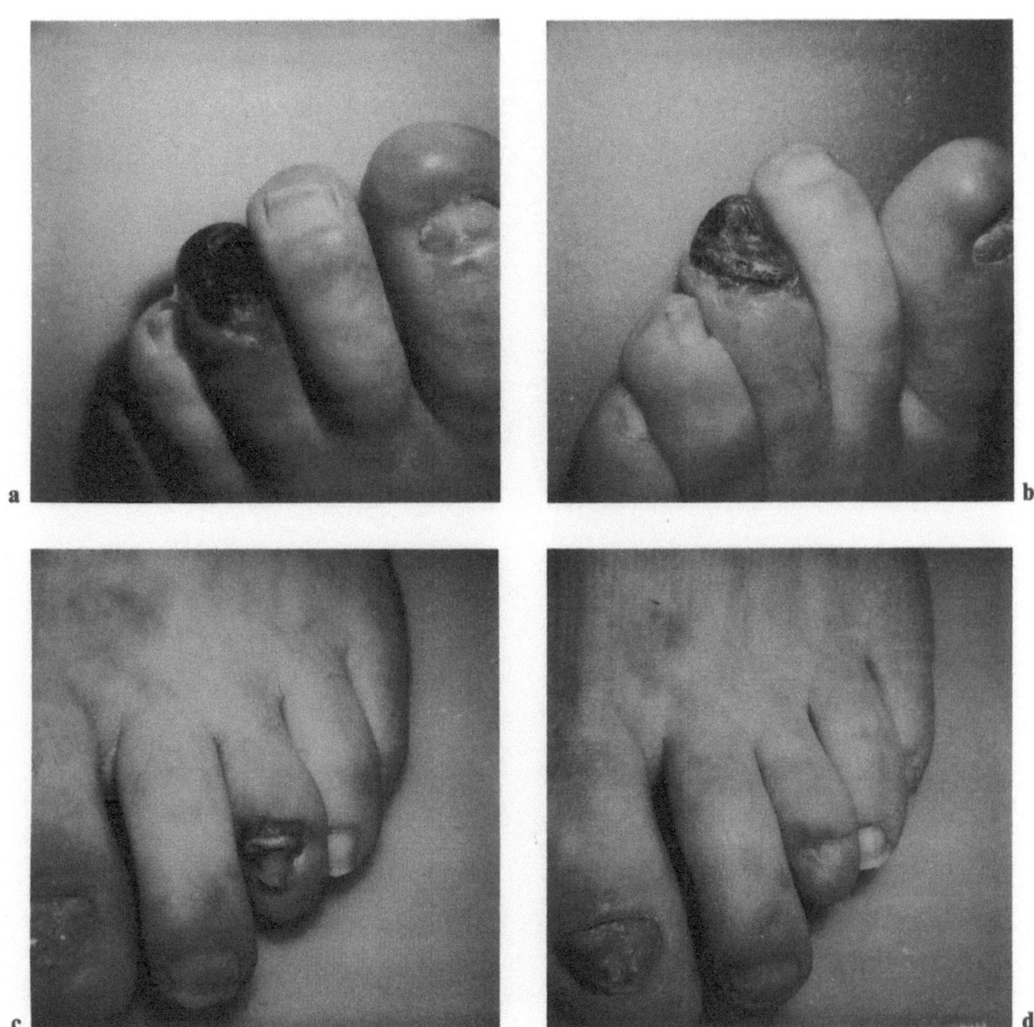

**Fig. 4a–d.** Man, aged 55, with gangrene of the left 1st and 3rd toes for which amputation of the left leg had been advised. The left foot before (**a**) and after treatment for 1 month (**b**), 2 months (**c**), and 3 months (**d**)

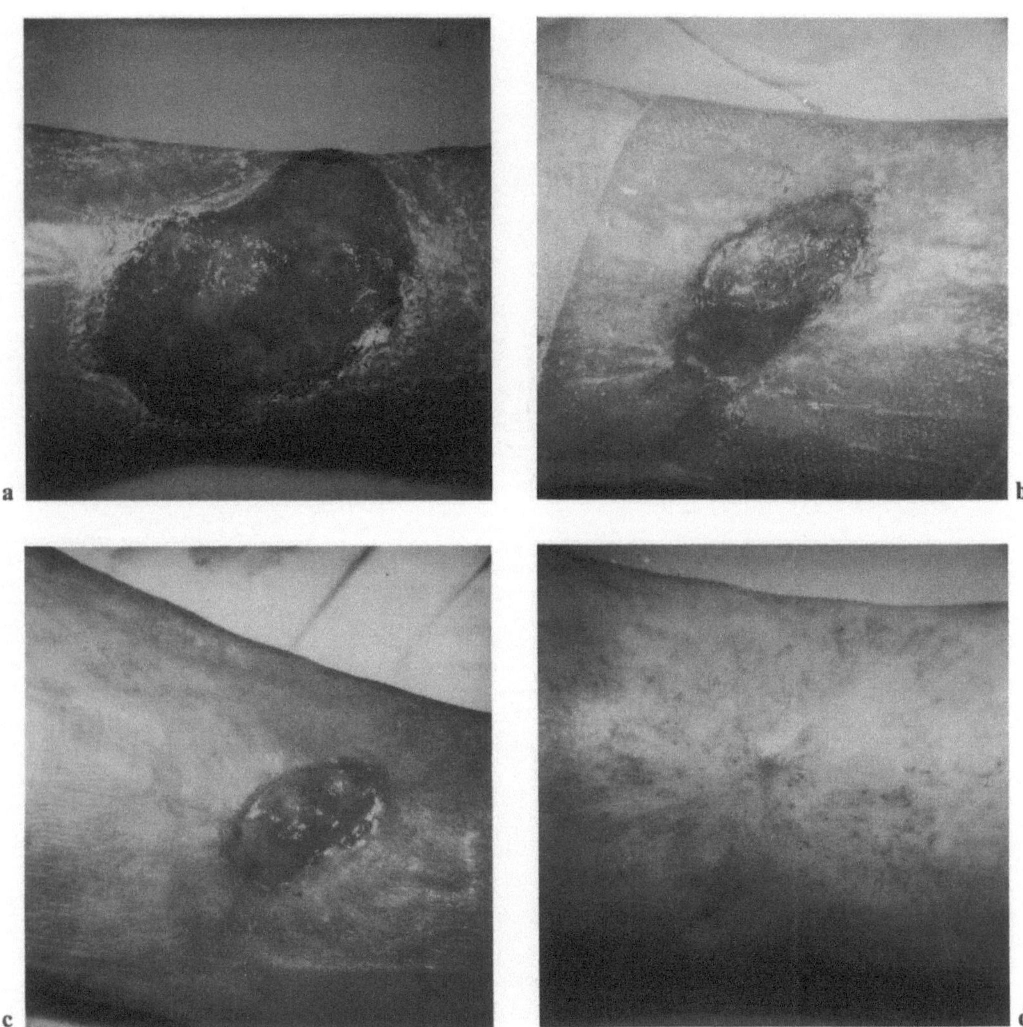

**Fig. 5a–d.** Woman, aged 71, with ischemic ulcers of the medial side of both calves. Diagnosed in a university clinic as "arteriosclerosis of both lower limbs and confirmed by arteriography to involve both common iliac and femoral vessels. Amputation of left leg was advised. Left leg before (**a**) and after treatment for 2 months (**b**), 3 months (**c**), and 8 months (**d**)

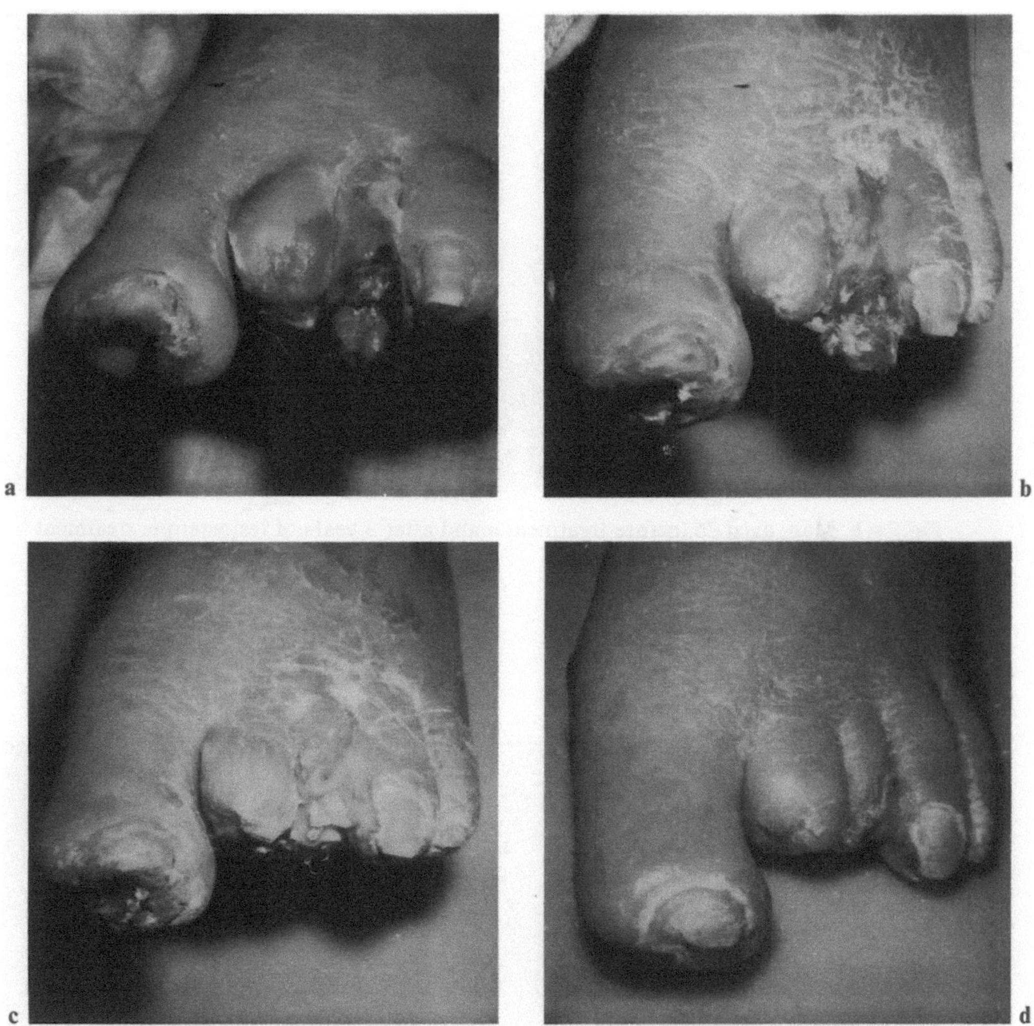

**Fig. 6a–d.** Man, aged 77, with gangrene of all 5 toes. **a** Before treatment, **b** after 3 weeks, **c** after 1 month, and **d** after 3 months. Ulceration healed completely

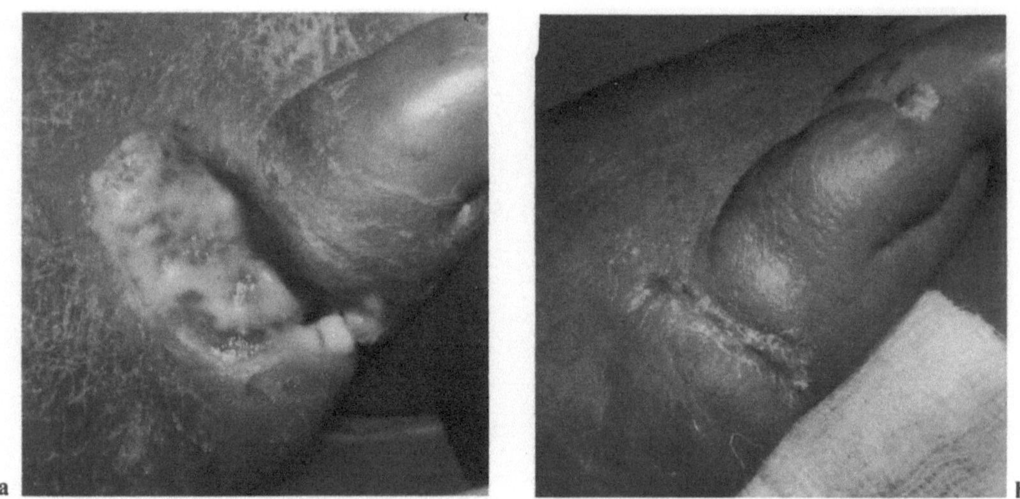

**Fig. 7 a, b.** Man, aged 76, before treatment **a** and after 3 years of testosterone treatment **b**

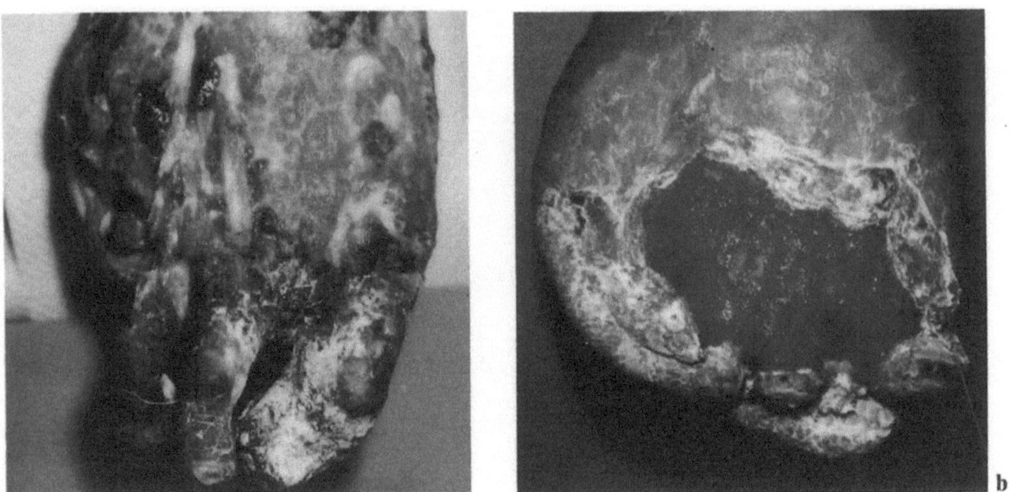

**Fig. 8 a, b.** Man, aged 44, before treatment **a** and after 14 months of treatment **b**. After a further 3 years of continuous treatment the gangrene healed completely

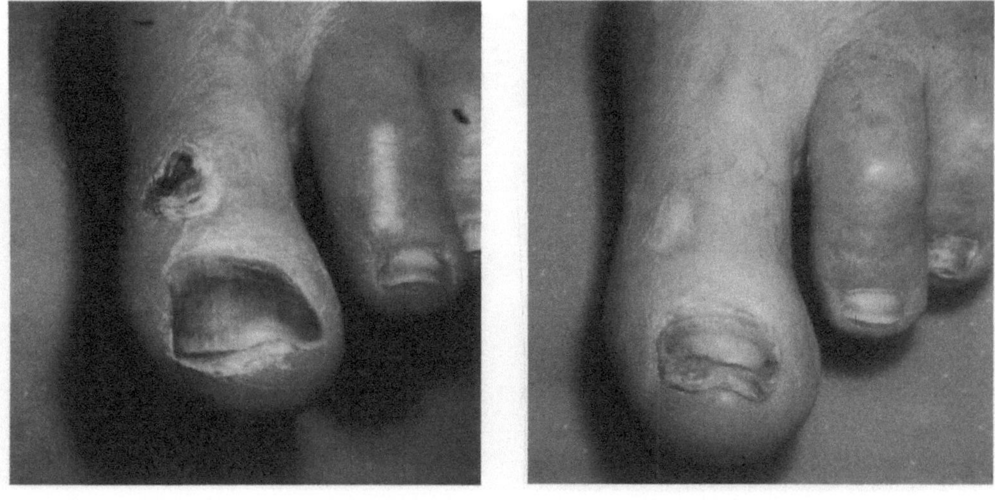

**Fig. 9 a, b.** Man, aged 76. before treatment **a** and after 8 months of treatment **b**

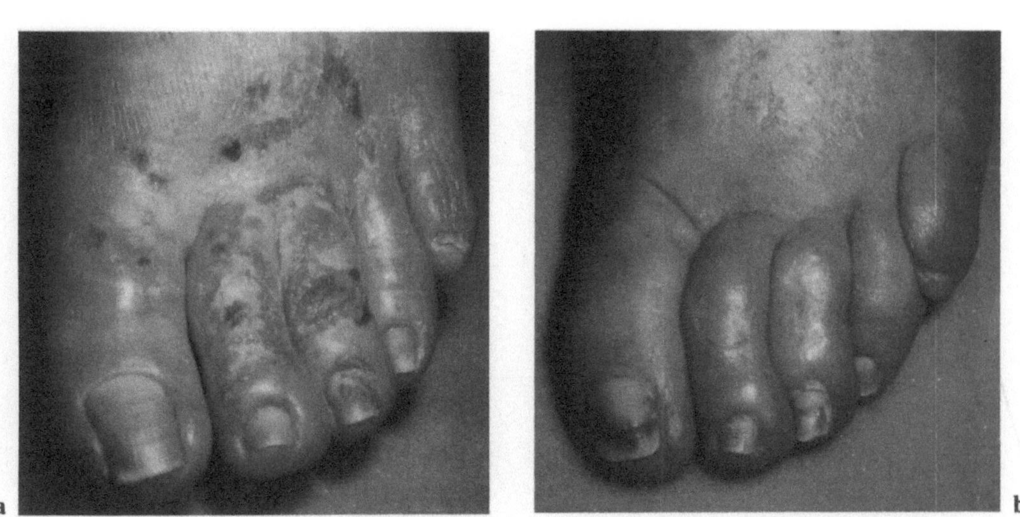

**Fig. 10 a, b.** Diabetic woman, aged 85, before treatment **a** and after 1 year of treatment **b**

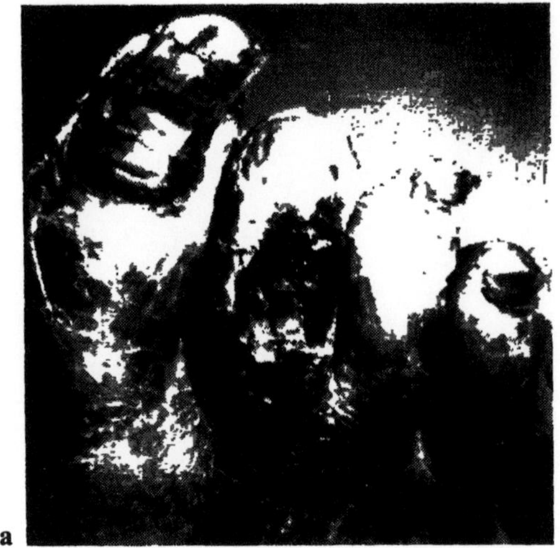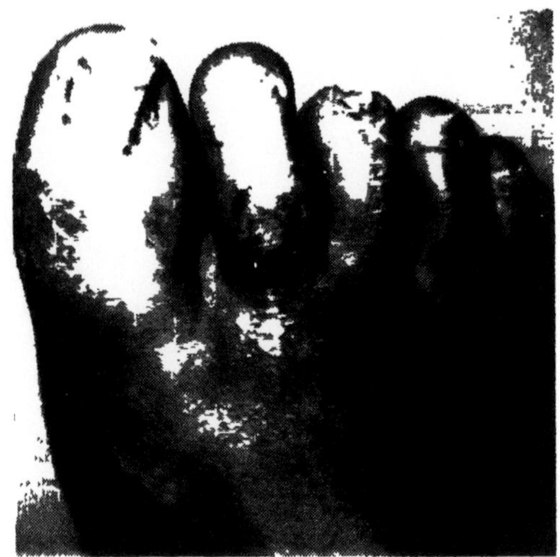

**Fig. 11 a, b.** Man, aged 57, before treatment **a** and after 5 months of treatment **b**. Gangrene had developed after sympathectomy

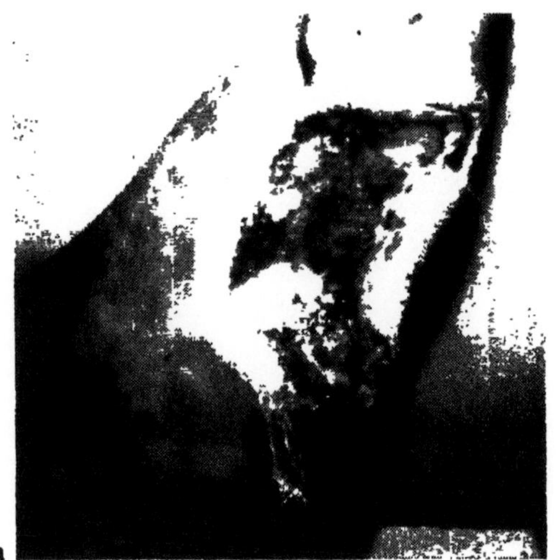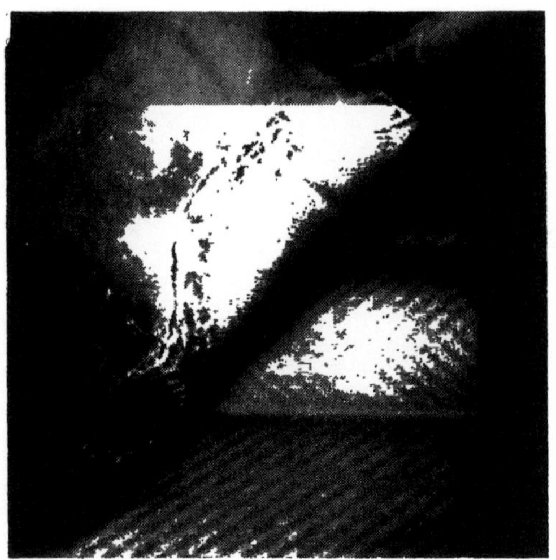

**Fig. 12 a, b.** Diabetic man, aged 77, before treatment **a** and after 8 months of testosterone treatment **b**

# Summary of Biochemical Aspects Relating to CVD

It is important to bear in mind that the problems posed by CVD are quite different from those associated with a specific metabolic endocrinological disease with a single etiology. Myxedema, for example, is a simple clinical case; by administrating thyroid hormone the patient can be considered to be cured. In CVD, however, we are not dealing with *a* single part of the metabolism; it refers to a larger and wider aspect, namely, all the different processes producing energy to maintain life itself, processes which are altered because of an oxygen deficiency.

I recall from my discussions with Professor Sir Hans Krebs, the Nobel Prize winner from the University of Oxford, that he warned me against speculation and philosophy. Yet he did not deny that great advances cannot be made without speculating and philosophizing, with subsequent scientific proof. Furthermore, he wrote to me,

I feel that your *clinical findings can stand for themselves* and do not necessarily need underpinning as far as practical medicine is concerned. After all, there are many methods of treatment which have no adequate biochemical foundation but are firmly based on clinical experience. I take it that you are anxious to see your clinical results and their interpretation *be underpinned by biochemical concepts, bearing in mind that all physiological and pathological events have some biochemical basis.*

It is therefore appropriate to follow the idea of Sir Hans Krebs and investigate the relationship between the theories put forward in this book concerning normal and pathological circulation with regard to metabolic biochemistry, and hence to estimate which measures and means can be used to normalize the basic metabolic disturbances of CVD. The following biochemical material is based primarily on medical textbooks and, in a few cases, on scientific publications.

## Metabolic Biochemistry

### Aerobic Metabolism

Under normal conditions pyruvic acid is oxidized in the Krebs cycle. Pyruvic acid is converted first to acetyl Co-A, which then combines with oxaloacetic acid to form citric acid. The conversion of citric acid to $\alpha$-ketoglutaric acid to succinic acid and back to oxaloacetic acid (via numerous intermediaries) results in the formation of two molecules of carbon dioxide and two molecules of water from each molecule of pyruvic acid. Altogether about forty molecules of the high-energy substance ATP are synthesized from every glucose molecule broken down by aerobic dissimilation (Green 1976, p. 112). Most carbohydrates and fats are converted completely in this way, and those amino acids not used in protein synthesis follow the same metabolic pathway. Such metabolism exhibits a general equilibrium between anabolic and catabolic processes.

## Anaerobic Metabolism

Anaerobic metabolism refers to the predominance of catabolic processes. Oxygen deficiency leads to an increase in catecholamines (Keele and Neil 1961, p. 124). This fact is, to a large degree, the basis of my theories. Catecholamines (adrenaline) cause, "by stimulating adenyl cyclase, an activation of phosphorylase in the liver and skeletal muscle. The consequences of this activation are a rise in the blood glucose and lactic acid levels" (and a lowering of pH) (Ganong 1975, p. 210; see also Keele et al. 1982, p. 416). Sympathetic overactivity decreases the efficiency of oxygen utilization. This, in turn, leads to an insufficient oxygen supply to meet the requirements for normal metabolism in the cell and *may lead to necrosis* (gangrene, infarct), with a contributory cause being the lowering of pH which may lead to a decrease in enzyme activities (Green 1976, p. 92). Decreased oxidation of coenzymes (NADH and FADH) under anaerobic conditions also inhibits the metabolic processes of the Krebs cycle.

All of these altered conditions may lead to a catastrophic drop in ATP. "The reduction of contractility (in the heart) is due to a deficient concentration of ATP. Such a situation is seen in hypoxia or ischaemia" (Keele et al. 1982, p. 137). With regard to the consequences of catecholamine excess Gilman et al. (1980) report that "large or repeated doses of epinephrine or other sympatomimetic amines given to experimental animals lead to damage of the *arterial wall* and *myocardium* so severe as to cause the appearance of necrotic areas, indistinguishable in the heart from myocardial infarcts." The fact referred to in this quotation might support the proposition that thrombosis and infarction have a common origin in the overproduction of catecholamines, and explain why infarction can occur independently of thrombosis. It is very interesting that the cells of arterial walls are affected in the same way by catecholamines (e.g., thrombosis).

Increased production of catecholamines increases the heart rate, which means a decrease in stroke volume for any given cardiac output; this may lead to oxygen deficiency.

$$Heart\ rate \times stroke\ volume = cardiac\ output$$

As reported in *Samson Wright's Applied Physiology* (Keele et al. 1982, p. 111), *"The higher the heart rate, the greater the myocardial oxygen usage for any given cardiac output."* And: "Increasing the stroke volume against a constant pressure (heart rate kept constant) does not greatly increase the myocardial $O_2$ usage, hence efficiency rises in a striking fashion." Furthermore, concerning the regulation of stroke volume we can read in *Best and Taylor's Physiological Basis of Medical Practice* (Brobeck 1979, p. 3–46) that "insulin and male hormones influence the hypertrophic response to mechanical overload."

## Double Effect of Catecholamines

Almost all claudication patients reveal that their claudication symptoms started at approximately the same time as they experienced impotence and/or lack of erection. Statistics show that especially the pelvic arteries of these patients are occluded by thrombi. This fact means decreased blood flow to the testicles and consequently decreased testosterone production. Furthermore, catecholamines themselves have recently been shown to counteract the production of these hormones. Thus catecholamines act in several ways, two of which are described above.

## Cholesterol

In current discussions of CVD the main issue is the problem of an increased cholesterol level. This assertion has been shown to be completely absurd. Oxygen deficiency leads to an insufficient amount of oxaloacetic acid for the oxidation of acetyl Co-A. These highly reactive 2C fragments cannot accumulate, resulting in an increase in the cholesterol level.

As I have emphasized so often before, the parameters involved in circulatory function are interrelated and interdependent. I imagine it as a mechanism consisting of a series of cogwheels, each wheel representing catabolic and anabolic parameters, which may be in a state of balance. Each wheel or rather parameter is dependent on all the others; in order to maintain homeostasis the system must adjust to the demands placed on it by its surroundings by sometimes increasing sympathetic tone and sometimes increasing parasympathetic tone. Testosterone affects all anaerobic disorders.

The attempts to affect one parameter isolated from the others demonstrate the ineffectiveness of such an approach. For example, a lot of effort has been placed in attempts to decrease the elevated cholesterol levels of CVD patients, often with fatal results. It is correct to say that raised cholesterol levels are a sign of a metabolic state unfavorable for the circulation, but this only means that cholesterol (like impaired carbohydrate metabolism, decreased fibrinolytic activity etc.) is an indicator of impaired circulation which should only be corrected indirectly by affecting *all* the parameters. Testosterone corrects all the parameters. It is incorrect to class cholesterol as a poisonous substance which, to some extent, must be removed from the body. Cholesterol is a vital substance; it is a precursor of androgens, estrogens, and cortisol among other substances. The fact that it has been singled out for treatment without considering the other parameters is explanation enough for the tragic results this approach has produced.

Testosterone administration can turn anaerobic metabolism into aerobic metabolism with the result that there is a decrease in the cholesterol level and, by improving the decreased glucose tolerance seen in CVD, the production of sufficient oxaloacetic acid for the oxidation of acetyl Co-A.

## Glucostat

The balance between cortisol (and catecholamines) and insulin is necessary for normal carbohydrate metabolism (Keele et al. 1982, p. 532). Oxygen deficiency leads to an increase in catecholamines (Keele and Neil 1961, p. 124). The oxygen deficiency seen in CVD causes impaired carbohydrate metabolism, which is a clinical sign in CVD patients.

– Both cortisol and catecholamine excess produces hyperglycemia.
– Secretion of adrenaline is stimulated by hypoglycemia.

In this sense adrenaline is antagonistic to the effects of insulin on the blood glucose level (Keele and Neil 1961, p. 442). As Keele et al. (1982, p. 532) phrase it,

"The release of glucose from glycogen by adrenaline or glucagon *depends on the 'permissive' presence of cortisol."* Thus adrenaline and cortisol have similar effects on the glucostat. Another major textbook, *Human Physiology* edited by Schmidt and Thews (see Brück 1983, p. 682), describes this in the following way: "Stress reactions involve not only the release of noradrenaline but also an increase in the rate of secretion of the *glucocorticoids* and of thyroxin."

### Shift from Anaerobic to Aerobic Metabolism or from Catabolic to Anabolic Processes

The biological effects of testosterone are so far reaching and complex that they are best illustrated by a consideration of not only the normal specific sexual effect, but also the ability of testosterone to shift anaerobic to aerobic metabolism.
Cortisol (and catecholamine) excess raises blood lipids and the plasma cholesterol level. This leads to atherosclerosis (CVD) (Keele et al. 1982, p. 532). This catabolic process is anabolically affected by the decrease in the cholesterol level by testosterone.
It is a quite natural reaction to get the impression that catabolic processes can be counteracted by administering anabolic substances. *Cortisol breaks down protein; testosterone builds up protein.* Or as Keele et al. (1982, p. 532) put it: "Cortisol promotes catabolism of proteins. Normally the breakdown of protein is counterbalanced by anabolic processes." These very important statements explain the underlying reasons for all the positive effects that testosterone has on CVD and anaerobic metabolism; namely, it decreases cholesterol and controls impaired carbohydrate metabolism. Therefore, I have pursued this idea by treating CVD patients with substances (e.g., testosterone) promoting *anabolic processes* with the positive results mentioned in this book. The fact that anabolic testosterone plays a definite role in the synthesis of protein, increasing all classes of RNA (see Brobeck 1979, p. 7–104), may explain how testosterone affects the activity of insulin (a polypeptide hormone), the action of which decreases the plasma glucose level and promotes aerobic metabolism. Furthermore, anabolic steroids are used clinically with success to minimize the serious catabolic side effects in patients treated with cortison preparations.
With ageing there is a tendency toward anaerobic metabolism, which correlates with line a in Fig. 1. It also agrees with the statement by Keele et al. (1982, p. 528), "It is often difficult to say whether degenerative changes are physiological or pathological in nature, but predisposition to fatal infections malignant disease and *cardiovascular catastrophes* accounts for the vast majority of deaths in old people." It is a fact that there is impairment, to a greater or lesser degree, of carbohydrate metabolism, demonstrated by the glucose tolerance test, in both the elderly and CVD patients. In both groups there is decreased oxygen utilization. Similarly, the corticoid-ketosteroid ratio increases in CVD and with ageing and the hexosamine-collagen ratio is decreased in both groups.


### Basis for Reliable Statistics

I believe that I have treated this subject in such a way that interested colleagues or scientists who have specialized in this field may be inspired to probe further into these problems. I have given powerful weapons to my colleagues, which will enable them to carry out reliable research on the basis of the metabolic alterations in the patients before and after treatment and on the effect of testosterone on these alterations. Here we are talking about known factors which can be evaluated statistically in contrast to those calculations which make use of far too many *unknown* and completely unreliable factors. The results that have been achieved by the use of testosterone instead of, for instance, amputations have naturally made a great impression and been discussed in medical literature all over the world with the result that CVD patients are now being examined before and after treatment, in the way that I have suggested, using reliable factors for statistics.

The facts which can be measured and statistically evaluated are:

1. Under anaerobic conditions the activity of dehydrogenating enzymes is decreased. Testosterone is necessary in reactivating these enzymes (proteins). At the University of Roskilde, Denmark, testosterone was used to raise the decreased level of the dehydrogenases of Krebs cycle in CVD patients.
2. Testosterone increases fibrinolytic activity (see, for example, World Health Organization 1972), which promotes oxygen uptake in tissue by increasing the hexosamine-collagen ratio (Pincus 1958).
3. Testosterone increases 2,3-diphosphoglycerate, thereby counteracting hypoxia (Ganong 1975, p. 489).
4. Gangrene, which is caused by hypoxia, is healed by the administration of testosterone.
5. Testosterone tends to reduce the risk of cardiac infarction and to normalize the other signs of oxygen deficiency which can be recognized on an ECG, resulting in milder and fewer attacks of angina pectoris, which often eventually disappear.
6. Testosterone can be used to normalize impaired carbohydrate metabolism.
7. Testosterone lowers the cholesterol level.

To investigate the role to testosterone in relation to regulation of carbohydrate metabolism where it decreases the cholesterol level, a study (mentioned in the first EOCCD Bulletin) was carried out by the state hospital in Copenhagen in which 300 CVD patients were treated with testosterone. The cholesterol concentration in blood fell during treatment to an average of 74% of the concentration before treatment. Much similar research has been carried out on this subject and published in leading medical journals.

## Resume

CVD is characterized by hypoxia leading to increased catecholamine production, hyperglycemia, impaired carbohydrate metabolism, excess of acetyl Co-A and hence increased cholesterol level. Cortisol and catecholamines are anti-insulin hormones. The primary characteristics of testosterone are that it increases 2,3-DPG (shift from anaerobic to aerobic metabolism), increases fibrinolytic activity (shift from anaerobic to aerobic metabolism), decreases the cholesterol level, and counteracts the impairment of carbohydrate metabolism which may result when cortisol breaks down protein to amino acids, producing glucose which may lead to hyperglycemia.

Incidentally, most of the biochemical material has been taken from *Samson Wright's Applied Physiology,* and with its help I have endeavored to provide a scientific basis for the testosterone treatment of CVD. I succeeded in arranging a meeting with the editor-in-chief of this textbook, Professor Eric Neil, just before this manuscript was to be printed. Professor Neil took the time to carefully read the first draft of this biochemical summary. He fully accepted its contents when I asked him directly whether my interpretation was correct or not. Furthermore, by recommending the insertion of the following references to the *Handbook of Physiology* in order to make my theories even more evident, he demonstrated that he had really grasped and agreed with the essence of my interpretation of the biological mechanisms of CVD:

1. Comparison of age and venous plasma norepinephrine (NE) in man:

   | Age | Plasma NE (ng/ml) |
   | --- | --- |
   | 20–29 | 0.266 |
   | 60–68 | 0.350 |

2. Influence of pH on catecholamine output of dog adrenal gland perfused with blood:

   | pH | Total catecholamine output (ng/gland per min) |
   | --- | --- |
   | 7.41 | 70 |
   | 6.84 | 532 |

3. Plasma catecholamines in myocardial infarction:

   | Mortality (n) | Plasma catecholamines (ng/ml) | |
   | --- | --- | --- |
   | | Epinephrine | Norepinephrine |
   | 7 of 9 | 0.27 | 4.1 |
   | 2 of 8 | 0.12 | 1.5 |
   | 1 of 8 | 0.09 | 0.61 |

4. Nicotine in tobacco smoke given to human subjects results in increases in the level of plasma catecholamines.

5. Hypoxia is a powerful stimuli causing the release of adrenal medullary hormones.

6. "Catecholamines inhibit release of insulin from the pancreas."

(Points 1–5 are from Callingham 1975, pp. 430, 433, 435, 436, and 438, respectively. Point 6 is from Moran 1975, p. 456.)

My English colleague Dr. Malcolm Carruthers, world known specialist for the autonomic nervous system, participated in a more detailed discussion with Professor Neil and described his conception in a letter to me. It reads in part:

He [Professor Neil] confirmed that the quotations that you used from Samson Wright's textbook of physiology, of which he had been Senior Editor for over 20 years, had been correctly interpreted and provided strong support for your arguments on the importance of anabolic steroids in CVD. As well as expressing interest in and general agreement with the lines of reasoning in the biochemical section of your book, he was kind enough to put us in toubh with another old colleague of mine in the Courtauld Institute of Biochemistry, Dr. William Coulson, Professor of Steroid Endocrinology, who was also positive and supportive in his views.

# Epilogue

The manuscript of this book is now finished. Sitting here, holding it in my hands, I have time to reflect on its theme, realizing that it may have been drowned in the flood of details that have been discussed. I will therefore repeat, in a brief and concentrated form, the reasons which prompted me to write it. First and foremost are the positive results achieved by testosterone treatment of CVD; the second important aspect is the scientific explanation of these results. Noted scientists who are familiar with these results consider my achievements to be exceptional in their importance for the "benefit of mankind," and others maintain that I have "solved the problem of CVD." All this is, of course, very gratifying and encouraging, but *personally* I am unable to accept this glorification.

At the beginning of this book the reader's attention was drawn to a number of doctors and scientists who achieved the same positive results that I have, but whose names have long since been forgotten the problem of CVD did not exist to the same extent it does today. They did not have, as I did, the possibility of underpinning their treatment scientifically by referring to valuable studies based on the most recent technical advances.

The huge patient material which it has been my lot to treat resulted in my becoming a central figure in this field. Naturally enough, my use of testosterone became the object of some discussion in which demands have persistently been raised that clinical trials be conducted, in particular those based on statistics, before testosterone therapy could be accepted.

In the Preface I touched upon the difficulties that would arise in the writing of this book if I would have followed the rules that apply for an ordinary scientific paper. This would have been impossible because, as I have claimed again and again, I have not looked on CVD as a disease in the usual sense of the word. My approach is scientific, based on facts from biology, biochemistry, and physiology, as opposed to the approach of those whose authority dominates the medical world for the time being, which has resulted in a confusion of groundless suppositions bordering on the outrageous. The uncertainty surrounding the CVD problem has given them the chance to spread their terror campaigns and create a meaningless guilt complex regarding life-style and diet. However, a worldwide wave of severe criticism seems to be rising against this authoritative attitude and all the theories and projects carried out in its wake.

I can, for instance, refer again to the article by Professor Oliver (1983) (see p. 38). From my correspondence with university officials in the United States I can quote the following about MRFIT: The authors of this report "knew, before they started, the multiple treatments would not work. They have squandered money, time and people," says one letter; and from another: "The diet-heart issue is very confused here now, since MRFIT was reported in September as a complete failure. That trial over ten years spent something like 114 million dollars, and so people are beginning to take a harder look at their persistence with this unrewarding preposition."

In his book (1978) on the cholesterol neurosis Hermann Mohler wrote: "The dietary dogma was a money-maker for segments of the food industry, a fund raiser for the Heart Association and busy work for thousands of fat-chemists." The explanation why they have been able to get away with their beguiling humbug must be that as definition of CVD has never been formulated. There has only been muddle.

Here it would be appropriate to quote Raab (1972 a) once again, who elaborates on this confusion.

Regardless of the variously reported nonexistence of thrombi and vascular occlusion in up to more than 50% of myocardial so-called infarctions, and regardless of frequent gross discrepancies between the incidence, degree and location of coronary vascular vs. myocardial structural lesions, such terms as "coronary occlusion", "coronary thrombosis", "coronary atherosclerosis", "coronary heart disease", "coronary artery disease" or plainly a "coronary" are indiscriminately and interchangeably used in clinical practice and *textbooks* and, especially, in *epidemiologic reports*. Unfortunately, some of the latter, in referring to nonautopsied patient material, glibly employ the terms "athersclerotic heart disease" or "occlusive coronary disease" or "atherosclerosis", *without any clear proof of the presence or absence of arterial occlusion, or of the degree and actual pathogenic involvement and significance of existing coronary lesions in the individual instances for statistical evaluation.*

Research must concentrate on the theories presented in this book, which are supported by fundamental medical thought as expressed in university textbooks. Let us start with *Samson Wright's Applied Physiology* (Keele and Neil 1969): "It is now becoming evident that the findings of cytology are of outstanding significance to both physiology, pathology and hence to *practical medicine*." This is exactly what I have made a special point of.

In *Medicinsk Kompendium* (Thaysen et al. 1975), which is the authorized textbook at several Scandinavian universities, we can read:

The mobilization of fatty acids from fatty tissue is stimulated by sympaticus (the sympathetic nervous system), circulating catecholamines, and many other hormones, and is inhibited by insulin and glucose (p. 1469).
The increased concentration of catecholamines inhibits the insulin production by pheochromocytom (p. 1401). [Concerning anomalies in fat metabolism] Both cholesterol and triglyceride are increased in plasma. There is often glucose intolerance (p. 1482).
Insulin is produced by proinsulin which is synthesized via the ribosomes RNA (p. 1399).
The complex of dehydrotestosterone and a receptor protein are presumed to penetrate the nucleus and cause the formation of RNA, resulting in protein synthesis (p. 1283).

The last point is in conformity with the previously mentioned passage in *Best and Taylor's Physiological Basis of Medical Practice* (Bardin 1979), which also deals with the androgen receptor complex "causing increased transfer of RNA to cytoplasm which results in protein synthesis, cellular growth and differentiated function" (pp. 7–104).

In Ganong's *Review of Medical Physiology* (1975, p. 210) we can read that, "by stimulating adenylate cyclase, epinephrine causes activation of the phosphorylase in liver and skeletal muscle. The consequences of this activation are a rise in the blood glucose and lactic acid levels." Gilman et al. (1980) report in *The Pharmacological Basis of Therapeutics* that "large or repeated doses of epinephrine or

other sympathomimetic amines given to experimental animals lead to damage to arterial walls and myocardium so severe as to cause the appearance of necrotic areas, indistinguishable in the heart from myocardial infarcts."
These fragments from textbooks are pieces of a mosaic which I have put together, and which form the basis of my theories. Can it be true that no one else has perceived the relationship between these fragments and the problem of CVD? I feel that one of the most convincing details in this book is the report that glucose tolerance is improved concurrently with dissimilation of fats after the administration of testosterone to CVD patients. Another detail which at least I find very convincing is the report by Sobel and Marmorston (1958) that androgens increase the H-C ratio, once again confirming that testosterone counteracts anaerobic metabolism.
The foundation upon which the entire medical profession is built, on which we act, discuss, think, talk, and treat our patients, is also the foundation on which the theories presented in this book are based. It is amazing and unbelievable that this foundation has had to give way, at least for a while, to theories which emphasize statistical surveys but are detached from the reality of treating patients. The only indisputable fact ist that any form of research must have as its only and final goal the ability to produce positive results in the treatment of patients. In this book I have pointed out that the only "solution" for CVD to date is provided by anabolic steroids that *can* produce positive results and help for patients.
Every politician, doctor, and layman who is a member of the EOCCD will press this case until the ineffective treatment of CVD has been replaced by that help which the leading authorities referred to in this book have suggested. It would be a great leap forward for mankind if testosterone treatment were accepted.
Where statistics are concerned in connection with CVD, I share the same doubts that many others have, and I repeat that statistical unreliability is due to the many unknown factors. The patient's own subjective testimony cannot be used scientifically. However, as I have said before, it is immensely difficult to assess the circulatory condition of a patient. Death can even overtake the man who has been termed perfectly healthy with regard to his circulation. This must be due to an as yet unknown factor. At the same time, a patient with an apparently hopeless circulatory condition, who has had extensive gangrenous areas that have healed, can enjoy life as if nothing were wrong with his circulation.
Increased cholesterol levels, hypertension, impaired carbohydrate metabolism, increased level of FFA, and ECG abnormalities are the factors which prove that we are indeed dealing with patients with circulatory disturbances. If testosterone treatment results in a normalization of these laboratory findings, we have objective signs of improvement in CVD patients. As far as I can judge, better scientific proof cannot be obtained for any disease.
With the knowledge acquired from such great patient material throughout so many years, I am convinced that those of my colleagues who institute clinical trials will sooner or later admit the positive effects of testosterone and will find it a waste of time to continue these investigations. I hope that my endeavors may act as an earnest appeal to my colleagues and to the editors of the medical publications, to climb up the sides of the pyramid and meet me at the summit. They will then realize that, when all of our individual efforts are pieced together, we

have a clear picture of CVD and its treatment with testosterone, and we have solved a vast problem "for the benefit of mankind."

I have called this final section an epilogue. Now, laying the book aside, I wonder where and how I fit into this discussion or dispute, and I thank the Lord that I have not supported the above-mentioned dominating "scientists" and that it has not been my fate to defend their standpoints and their "science."

# Abstracts

The following references are given with abstracts (quotations) and pertinent comments. Some of them have already been used in the text.


Raab W (1969) Pathological fundamentals of the origin and prevention of degenerative heart disease. Ann NY Acad Sci 156:281–284


*Abstract.* For 50 years a mechanistic interpretation of hypoxic degenerative heart disease prevailed as being merely a problem of vascular oxygen supply to the heart muscle. Hardly any attention was paid to the fact that vital oxygen availability to the myocardial tissue depends not only on vascular oxygen supply but also on metabolic oxygen consumption by the myocardial tissue. Any major discrepancy between these two logically inseparable factors is bound to create local hypoxia and to result in functional and structural alterations that are, in turn, largely mediated by derangements in the cellular electrolyte balance.

*Comment.* In this publication Raab points out that if there is insufficient oxygen to meet the metabolic requirements of the cell anaerobic metabolism arises. In the text I have given numerous examples supporting Raab's theories. As a result of this alteration a chain of biochemical reactions occur, including interference with carbohydrate metabolism leading to accumulation of plasma lipids. This may explain the increased plasma cholesterol levels. The decrease in ATP with anaerobic metabolism means increased lactate and hydrogen ion ($H^+$) concentrations which cause a decrease in the activity of cellular enzymes.


Selye H (1969) La evolution del concepto del stress. Folia Clin Int 32:471–489


*Abstract.* Unlike the common myocardial infarcts described in textbooks, those elicited in animals after pretreatment with corticoids and sodium salts are not accompanied by vascular occlusion. It is clear that animal myocardial necroses can be produced without coronary obstruction, apparantly as a consequence of a direct interference within the cardiac muscle itself. It is also evident that these necroses can be prevented by chemical agents whicht act on the myocardium directly and not through improvement of its blood supply.

*Comment.* This resumé emphasizes again that CVD is not necessarily due to thrombosis and, as I point out in the text, stress hormones such as cortisol decrease sensitivity to insulin so that here again there is impaired glucose tolerance.
Selye is of the opinion that myocardial necrosis can occur without thrombosis; in this case the abnormality is not to be found in the vascular supply but within the cardiac muscle itself. Selye believes that this necrosis can be prevented by chemical substances which act on the myocardium directly and not on the blood supply. The medical literature shows this substance to be testosterone.


Selye H (1970 b) Stress and ageing. J Am Geriatr Soc 18:679–680


*Abstract.* It has always been assumed as self-evident that ageing has a specific cause and that we might discover what this is and perhaps find a way to block it. There is no justification for such an assumption. Undoubtedly, the hormones regulating growth and sexual development as well as numerous dietary, nervous and other factors play a decisive role in the process of growing up. Yet we have no reason to suspect that a unified theory of "the growing-up process" could be formulated or that, in this respect, the clock could be turned back by some panacea which would interfere with all the relevant biological reactions.

*Comment.* Here Selye remarks on the idea illustrated by curve in Fig. 1. We cannot prevent an individual ageing, or turn back the clock with some medication.

Raab W (1972 a) Why "Myocardiology". In: Bajusz E, Rona G (eds) Recent advances in studies on cardiac structure and metabolism, vol 1, Myocardiology. University Park Press, Baltimore pp 5–8

*Abstract.* Regardless of the variously reported nonexistence of thrombi and vascular occlusions in up to more than 50% of myocardial so-called infarctions, and regardless of frequent gross discrepancies between the incidence, degree and location of coronary vascular vs myocardial structural lesions, such terms as "coronary occlusion", "coronary thrombosis", "coronary atherosclerosis", "coronary heart disease", "coronary artery disease" or plainly "a coronary" are indiscriminately and interchangeably used in clinical practise and textbooks, and especially in epidemiological reports...
Profound, potentially pathogenic, and mutually aggravating influences of sympatho-adrenal catecholamines and of adrenal corticoids upon the oxygen economy and electrolyte balance of the heart muscle have been intensively investigated over many years. This popular, but somewhat worn-out cliché for "coronary heart disease" may more appropriately be read as meaning "cardiac hypoxic dysionism" in keeping with present day knowledge and concepts.

*Comment.* I agree that it would be a good idea to adopt Raab's expression for circulatory disease "cardiac hypoxic dysionism" because it gives a description of the nature of the disease. How often have I heard medical students complain of confusion over the many different theories used to describe this problem.

Raab W (1972 b) Cardiotoxic effects of emotional, socioeconomic, and environmental stress. In: Bajusz E, Rona G (eds) Recent advances in studies on cardiac structure and metabolism, vol 1, Myocardiology. University Park Press, Baltimore, pp 707–713

*Abstract.* Today's literature suggests that, jointly with vascular oxygen-supply-limiting factors, centrally controlled neuroendocrine mechanisms dominate the myocardial pathogenesis. By interfering with myocardial oxygen economy (catecholamines) and carbohydrate metabolism (glucocorticoids), they derange vital myocardial electrolyte equilibrium (loss of K and Mg, gain in Na), thus disturbing stimulus formation and conduction, cell contractility and structure, largely under the influence of civilization-induced emotional and environmental stresses.

*Comment.* Here again Raab points out the poor oxygen economy in the myocardium caused by catecholamines and impaired glucose tolerance by cortisol and the subsequent derangement of myocardial electrolyte equilibrium.

Oyama T, Aoki N, Kudo T (1972) Effect of halothane anaesthesia and of surgery on plasma testosterone levels in man. Anesth Analg 51:130–133

*Abstract.* Levels of plasma testosterone in 14 male patients decreased during operation, the lowest being detected on the 1st postoperative day. The significant reduction of plasma testosterone levels continued for a week.

*Comment.* Here is a report of how the testosterone plasma level is influenced by stress. I can visualise that during an acute myocardial infarction there is a great increase in the catabolic processes and a decrease in normal metabolism such that the catabolic processes predominate and fatal necrosis occurs.

Allison SP, Prowse K, Chamberlain MJ (1967) Failure of insulin response to glucose load during operation and after myocardial infarction. Lancet I/292:478–481

*Abstract.* We report preliminary results suggesting that surgical operations are associated with failure of the insulin response to a glucose load, and that there is a similar failure in the first 12 hours after myocardial infarction. We suggest that this may be a nonspecific effect of stress, mediated by adrenaline.

*Comment.* I give numerous confirmations of these results in the text. We must appreciate the homeostasis between the catabolic and anabolic forces which occur throughout life. It is only when the catabolic processes gain control that problems arise. Allison compares the surgical patient's situation with that of myocardial infarction and suggests that the cause for the similarity can be found in catecholamines.

Allison SP, Tomlin PJ, Chamberlain MJ (1969) Some effects of anaesthesia and surgery on carbohydrate and fat metabolism. Br J Anaesth 41:588–593

*Abstract.* The emotional stress of being brought to the operating theatre and the stress of surgery seems to be more important than anaesthesia in causing a rise in blood sugar and plasma FFA. There was a corresponding fall in levels of plasma insulin. The clinical significance of this phenomenon rests on the fact that stress causes a temporary diabetic state.

*Comment.* Allison et al. point once again to the stress phenomenon during an operation as causing a rise in blood sugar and plasma free fatty acids with decreased plasma insulin. To use his own expression, stress causes a "temporary diabetic state." W. F. Ganong (1975) similarly states: "By stimulating adenylate cyclase, epinephrine causes activation of the phosphorylase in liver and skeletal muscle. The consequences of this activation are a rise in the blood glucose and lactic acid levels." Here we have another example of dysstress whereby the production of testosterone decreases as mentioned previously.

Winther O (1966) Exercise and blood-fibrinolysis. Lancet 291:1195–1196

*Abstract.* I report her a study to determine whether repeated physical training can induce sustained activation of blood fibrinolysis. In all persons except one, there was a clear shortening of the lysis-time during each exercise session, but there was no sustained effect.

Winther O (1965) Testosterone and fibrinolytic activity. Scand J Clin Lab Invst, Suppl. 99:207–210

*Abstract.* Testosterone was given as propionate in doses of 250 mg 3 times weekly intramuscularly. On a dose of 250 mg 3 times weekly the lysis time was within the normal range. Related to fibrinolysis, the dose of testosterone seems to be very important. In this case the critical dose was between 500 and 750 mg weekly; 250 mg 3 times weekly was started. Symptomatic improvement correlated clearly with increased, and deterioration with reduced fibrinolytic activity.

*Comment.* The articles by Dr. Winther have shown that physical activity and testosterone have similar effects. In this connection I would like to remind the reader about the WHO report from the symposium held in Madrid in 1972, already mentioned in the text.

Gudbjarnason S, Ravens KC, Mathes P (1976) Metabolic changes in infarcted and noninfarcted myocardium during the postinfarction period. Recent Adv Stud Card Struct Metabol 1:439–446

*Abstract.* Results suggest that diet and anabolic hormones may play an important role during tissue repair and muscle recovery following acute myocardial infarction. Treatment with anabolic steroids significantly increases the ATP levels of noninfarcted muscle. Scar formation in cardiac muscle is markedly reduced in animals treated with anabolic steroid and collagen formation is reduced by 26%.

*Comment.* Gudbjarnason et al. report an increase in ATP levels caused by treatment with anabolic steroids. This effect of testosterone is fundamental in the treatment of circulatory disease. The reduction in collagen is confirmed by Sobol and Marmorston (1958) (androgen increases the H-C ratio).

Ravens KG (1970) Der Einfluß von anabolen Hormonen und von Diät auf den myokardialen Gehalt an energiereichen Phosphaten während der Infarktheilung. Ver Dtsch Ges Kreisl-Forsch 36:314–319

*Abstract.* Administration of anabotic steroids significantly diminishes the reduction of ATP and creatine phosphate in non-infarcted tissue and stimulates recovery. This indicates a positive effect of anabolic agents upon the synthetic and mechanical functions of the heart muscle after artificial infarction in dogs.

*Comment*. Ravens once again confirms that anabolic steroids significantly decrease the reduction in ATP. This agrees entirely with the findings of Gudbjarnason et al.

Sufin G, Prutkin L (1974) Experimental diabetes and the response of the sex accessory organs of the castrate male rat to testosterone propionate. Invest Urol 11(5):361–369

*Abstract*. It was conluded that, although partial testosterone action is possible in the face of insulin deficiency, the presence of insulin is required for the full restorative effect of testosterone on the sex accessory tissue of the castrate male rat.

*Comment*. This is another example of the testosterone action in connecton with insulin.

Kochakian CD (1976) Regulation of tissue enzymes. In: Kochakian CD (ed) Anabolic-androgenic steroids. Springer, Berlin Heidelberg New York, pp 247–286 (Handbook of experimental pharmacology, vol 43)

*Abstract*. A large number of enzymes in several of the target tissues have been studied in an attempt to delineate the metabolic effects of testosterone and related compounds. Dose and duration of treatment, age, sex and nutritional status are contributing and modifying factors.

*Comment*. We recommend that this book be studied carefully; it documents the effect of testosterone, in agreement with many of the issues dealt with in this book.

Seliverstov SA (1969) The effect of nerobolon on the blood supply, cardiac activity, and haemodynamics. Farm Toksicol 32:59–62

*Abstract*. After an eight-day long administration of anabolic steroid, the arterial pressure was reduced, the systolic period shortened, the diastole lengthed, contractile capacity of the myocardium increased, and the mechanical efficiency of the heart increased without causing any substantial changes in the pulse rate and peripheral resistance.

*Comment*. This underlines the theories that anabolic steroids and physical training have the same beneficial influence on the circulation.

# References


Aakvaag A, Bentdal O, Quigstad K, Walstad P, Ronningen H, Fonnum F (1978) Testosterone and testosterone-binding globulin (TeBG) in young men during prolonged stress. Int J Androl 1:22–31

Albanese AA (1965) Never methodology in the clinical investigation of anabolic steroids. J New Drugs 5:108–224

Allison SP, Prowse K, Chamberlain MJ (1967) Failure of insulin response to glucose load during operation and after myocardial infarction. Lancet I/292:478–481

Allison SP, Tomlin PJ, Chamberlain MJ (1969) Some effects of anaesthesia and surgery on carbohydrate and fat metabolism. Br J Anaesth 41:588–593

Andersen P, Norman N, Hjermann, I (1983) Reduced fibrinolytic capacity associated with low ratio of serum testosterone to oestradiol in healthy coronary high-risk men. Scand J Haematol [Suppl 39] 30:53–57

Arndt H (1939) Zur Therapie extragenitaler Störungen mit Sexualhormonen. Wien Med Wochenschr 89:222–227

Atkinson J (1983) News from American hearts; 56 scientific sessions. Academy Newsletter 17 Nov 1983, p 8

Bardin W (1979) Hormonal control of testicular function. In: Brobeck JR (ed) Best and Taylor's physiological basis of medical practice, 10th edn. Williams and Wilkins, Baltimore

Bergamini E (1969) Additive effects of testosterone and insulin on glycogen content and 2-deoxyglucose phosphorylation in rat levator ani muscle. Biochem Biophys Acta (Amst) 177:235–240

Bergamini E, Bombara G, Pellegrino C (1969) The effect of testosterone on glycogen metabolism in rat levator ani muscle. Biochim Biophys Acta (Amst) 177:220–234

Bleha O, Küchel O (1967) Clinical endocrinology. SZN, Prague, pp 430–431

Boyd W (1965) Pathology for the physician, 7th edn. Lea and Febinger, Philadelphia

Brobeck JR (ed) (1979) Best and Taylor's physiological basis of medical practice, 10th edn. Williams and Wilkins, Baltimore

Bubenheim H (1953) Über die Angina pectoris und ihre Hormonbehandlung. Med Klin 44:1632–1634

Butenandt A (1934) Über die Physiologie und Chemie der Sexualhormone. Verh Dtsch Ges Inn Med 46:276–194

Callingham BA (1975) Catecholamines in blood. In: Blaschko H, Sayers G, Smith AD (eds) Endocrinology. American Physidogical Society, Washington DC, chap 28 (Handbook of physiology, sect 7, vol 6)

Carlson LA, Pernow B (1962) Studies on the peripheral circulation and metabolism in man. II. Oxygen utilisation and lactate pyruvate formation on the legs at rest and during exercise in patients with arteriosclerosis obliterans. Acta med Scand 171:311–323

Carruthers M (1980) Danish experience in the treatment of advanced circulatory disease with anabolic steroids. Bull EOCCD 6

Damber JE, Janson PO (1978) The effects of LH adrenaline and noradrenaline on testicular blood flow and plasma testosterone concentrations in anaesthetized rats. Acta Endocrinologica 88:390–396

Davidson JF, Lockhead M, McDonald GA, McNicol GP (1972) Fibrinolytic enhancement by stanozolol. A double blind trial. Br J Heamatol 22:543–559

Department of Health, Education and Welfare (1979) Healthy people: the surgeon general's report on health promotion and disease prevention. Government Printing Office, Washington, D.C.

Detweiler DK (1979) Circulation. In: Brobeck JR (ed) Best and Taylor's physiological basis of medical practise, 10th edn. Williams and Wilkins, Baltimore

Dingman JF, Linn NY (1963) Androgen metabolism in patients with hypercholesteremia and coronary artery disease. JAMA 186:316–320

Doyle AE (1983) What is ageing? Medicographia 5:

Edwards EA, Hamilton JB, Duntley SQ (1939) Testosterone propionate as a therapeutic agent in patients with organic diseases of the peripheral vessels. N Engl J Med 220:865

Edwards EA, Hamilton JB, Duntley SQ, Hubert G (1941) Cutaneous vascular and pigmentary changes in castrate and eunuchoid men. Endocrinology 28:119–128

Ehrlich JC, Shinohara Y (1964) Low incidence of coronary thrombosis in myocardial infarction. Arch Pathol 78:432–444

Einfeldt H (1970) Kredsløbssygdomme (Circulatory disease). Report 3, Danish Society for the Prevention of Circulatory Diseases, Copenhagen

Einfeldt H (1976) Zur Therapie von Durchblutungsstörungen mit Sexualhormonen und deren Derivaten. Therapiewoche 26:4111–4137

Fearnley GR (1962) Increase blood fibrinolytic activity by testosterone. Lancet I:128–132

Fiegel G (1961) Der Einfluß von anabolen Substanzen auf den Myokardstoffwechsel. Ihre Verwertung in der Behandlung von Herzmuskelschäden. Ärztl Forsch 15:310–317

Fiegel G (1962) Untersuchungen über die Wirkung von anabolen Substanzen bei chronisch-degenerativen Myokardschädigungen. Ärztl Forsch 16/3:74

Fiegel G, Kelling HW, Kukwa D (1962) Der reparative Effekt anaboler Steroide am geschädigten Myocard. Z Ärztl Fortbild 51:882–891

Franke H (1981) The heart in age. Ciba Rev 3

Fuller JH, Shipley MJ, Rose G, Jarrett RJ, Keen H (1980) Coronary heart disease risk and impaired glucose tolerance. Lancet I:1973–1976

Gall L (1970) Untersuchungen über den Fett- und Kohlenhydrat-Stoffwechsel beim Menschen unter Einfluß von 1-alpha-methyl-5-alpha-Andostan-17-beta-01-3-on. Dissertation, University of Würzburg

Ganong WF (ed) (1975) Review of medical physiology, 7th edn. Lange Medical Publications, Los Altos

Gillespie CA, Edgerton VR (1970) The role of testosterone in exercise-induced glycogen supercompensation. Horm Metab Res 2:364–366

Gilman AG, Goodman LS, Gilman A (eds) (1980) Goodman and Gilman's the pharmacological basis of therapeutics, 6th edn. McMillan, New York

Goldstein S (1978) Human genetic disorders that feature premature onset and accelerated pregression of biological ageing. In: Schneider EL (ed) The genetics of ageing. Plenum, New York

Gorokhovsky BI, Kitaeva II (1970) The use of anabolic hormones in myocardial infarction (in Russian). Klin Med (Mosk) 48:29–34

Green JH (1976) An introduction to human physiology, 4th edn. Oxford University Press, Oxford

Greenberg S, Heitz DC, Long JP (1973) Testosterone-induced depression of adrenergic activity in the perfused canine hindlimb. Proc Soc Exp Biol Med 142:883–888

Gudbjarnason S, Ravens KG, Mathes P (1972) Metabolic changes in infarcted and non-infarcted myocardium during the post infarction period. In: Bajusz E, Rona G (eds) Myocardiology. Urban and Schwarzenberg, München: University Park Press, Baltimore, pp 439–446 (Recent advances in studies on cardiac structure and metabolism, Vol. I)

Haan D (1963) Anabolic hormones in heart therapy. Angiology 14:449–450

Hamerski W (1974) Durabolin in the treatment of diabetic proliferative anginoretinopathy (in Russian). Klin Onczna 44/5:461–465

Hamilton JB, Hubert G (1938) Photographic nature of tanning of the human skin as shown by studies of male hormone therapy. Science 18:2290

Hammer F (1966) Zur Behandlung von Altersherzerkrankungen mit anabolen Steroiden. Med Welt 17:2814–2817

Harper AE (1980) Invited response to Congressman Richmond: another view of the politics of cholesterol. J Nutr Ed 12:187–188

Hazelwood RL, O'Brien KD (1961) Modification of glucagon-induced hyperglycemia in rats by 17-ethyl-19-nortestosterone. Proc Soc Exp Biol Med 106:851–854

Hedner U, Nilsson IM, Isacson S (1976) Effect of ethyloestrenol on fibrinolysis in the vessel wall. Br Med J 2:729–731

Holm J, Dahllöf AG, Björntorp P, Schersten T (1973) Enzyme studies in muscles of patients with intermittent claudication. Effects of training. J Clin Lab Invest [Suppl 128] 31:201–205

Hume DM, Bell CC, Bartter F (1962) Direct measurement of adrenal secretion during operative trauma and convalescence. Surgery 52/1:174–187

Jaffe MD (1977) Effect of testosterone cypionate on postexercise ST segment depression. Br Heart J 39:1217–1222

Janda J, Urbanová D, Mrhová O, Linhart J (1972) The effect of muscular work on the activities on certain enzymes in skeletal muscle in chronic muscular ischaemia. Cor Vasa 14:312–320

Janda J, Linhart J, Kasalický J (1974) Experimental chronic ischemia of skeletal muscle in rat. Physiol Bohemosl 23:521–526

Janda, J, Mrhová O, Urbanová D, Linhart J (1976) The effect of anabolic hormone 19-nortestosterone propionate on the metabolism of striated muscle during experimental ischemia. Pfluegers Arch 361:159–163

Jarret PE, Morland M, Clémenson G, Browse NL (1976) Treatment of Ranaud's syndrome with Stanozolol. Br J Surg 62:654

Johnson LC, O'Shea JP (1969) Anabolic steroids: effect on strength development. Science 164:957–959

Kalliomäki JL, Seppälä P (1963) Norandrostenolone decanoate as a cardiac anabolizer studied by means of electrocardiographic changes. Cardiologica 43:124–128

Keele CA, Neil E (1961) Samson Wright's applied physiology, 11th edn. Oxford University Press, Oxford

Keele CA, Neil E, Noel N (1982) Samson Wirght's applied physiology, 13 th edn. Oxford University Press, Oxford

Kochakian CD (1951) The effect of androgens on the metabolism. J Suisse Med 4:985–989

Kochakian CD (1976) Regulation of tissue enzymes. In: Kochakian CD (ed) Anabolic-androgenic steroids. Springer, Berlin Heidelberg New York, pp 247–286 (Handbook of experimental pharmacology, vol 43)

Koppelman J (1973) Skin and muscle flow during exercise in intermittent claudication. Scand J Clin Lab Invest [Suppl 128] 31:93–96

Krall LP (1970) Treatment of early diabetes. Adv Metab Disord [Suppl] 1:395

Kraus H, Raab W (1964) Krankheiten durch Bewegungsmangel. Barth, Munich

Krüger GAW (1969) Die therapeutische Beeinflussung von hormonmangelbedingten Herz- und Kreislaufstörungen durch Substitution mit einem synthetischen Androgen. Med Heute 18:16–19

Kutschera-Aichbergen H (1966) Anabolika bei biochemischen Myocardschäden. Wiener Med Wochenschr 16:352

Landon J, Wynn W, Houghton BJ, Cooke JNC (1962) Effect of methandienone on response to glucagon, adrenalin, and insulin in the fasted subject. Metabolism 11/5:513–523

Leonard S (1952) Effect of castration and testosterone propionate injection on glycogen storage in skeletal muscle. Endocrinology 51:293–297

Lesser MA (1946) Testosterone propionate therapy in one hundred cases of angina pectoris. J Clin Endocrinol 6:549–557

Meade T, Chakrabarti R, Haines AP, North WRS, Stirling Y (1979) Characteristics affecting fibrinolytic activity and plasma fibrogen concentrations. Br Med J 1:153–156

Meyer-Mölleringhof W (1964) Testosteron-Medikation beim Herzinfarkt. Med Welt 15:1631–1633

Møller J (1977 a) The concentration of cholesterol and testosterone in the blood of male patients with circulatory diseases. Bull EOCCD 1:1–4

Møller J (1977 b) Bull EOCCD 2:6–11

Mohler H (1978) Die Cholesterin-Neurose. Salk, Frankfurt

Molinari PE, Neri LL (1979) Effect of a single oral dose of oxymetholone on the metabolism of human erythrocytes. Exp Hematol 6:648–654

Moran NC (1975) Adrenergic receptors. In: Blaschko H, Sayers G, Smith AD (eds) Endocrinology. American Physiological Society, Washington DC, chap 29 (Handbook of physiology, sect 7, vol 6)

Multiple Risk Factor Intervention Trial Research Group (1982) Multiple Risk Factor Intervention Triol. JAMA 248:1465–1476

Neumann F (1977) Hormonale Regulation der Sexualdifferenzierung bei Säugetieren. Vorlesungsreihe Schering, Heft 3

Nikki P, Takki S, Tammisto T, Jäättela A (1972) Effect of operative stress on plasma catecholamine levels. Ann Clin Res 4:146–151

Oji N, Moriwaki T, Shigeta Y, Wada M (1960) Steroid hormones and diabetes mellitus. Med J Osaka 11:233

Okamoto R, Hatani M, Tsukitani M, Suehiro A (1983) The effect of oxygen on the development of atherosclerosis in WHHL rabbits. Atherosclerosis 47:47–53

Oliver MF (1981) Interview. Berlingske Tidende 15 Jan 1981

Oliver MF (1983) Should we not forget about mass control of coronary risk factors. Lancet II:37–38

Oppenheimer JR (1960) Science and common understanding (in Danish). Gyldendals Uglegøger, Copenhagen

Otter G (1960) The influence of anabolic substances on the nitrogen balance in surgical patients. Archivum Chir Neeri 12:496–504

Oyama T, Aoki N, Kudo T (1972) Effect of halothane anesthesia and of surgery on plasma testosterone levels in man. Anesth Analg 51/1:130–133

Parker JP, Bierne GJ, Desai JN et al. (1972) Androgen-induced increase in red-cell 2.3-diphosphoglycerate. N Engl J Med 287:381–382

Pernow B, Saltin B, Wahren J, Cronestrand R (1973) Muscle metabolism during exercise in patients with occlusive arterial disease; effect of reconstructive surgery. Scan J Clin Lab Invest [Suppl 128] 31:21–25

Phillips GB, Castelli WP, Abbott ED, McNamara PM (1983) Association of hyperestrogenemia and coronary heart disease in men in the Framingham cohort. Am J Med 74:863–869

Pincus G (ed) (1958) Recent progress in hormone research, vol 14. Academic, New York

Raab W (1949) Neurohormonalbedingte Herzkrankheiten. Pathogenese und Therapie. Arch Kreislaufforsch 15:39–63

Raab W (1969) Pathological fundamentals of the origin and prevention of degenerative heart disease. Ann NY Acad Sci 156:281–284

Raab W (1972a) Why myocardiology. In: Bajusz E, Rona G (eds) Myocardiology. University Park Press, Baltimore, Urban and Schwarzenberg, Munich, pp 5–8 (Recent advances in studies on cardiac structure and metabolism, vol 1)

Raab W (1972b) Cardiotoxic effects of emotional, socioeconomic, and environmental stress. In: Bajusz E, Rona G (eds) Myocardiology. University Park Press, Baltimore; Urban and Schwarzenberg, Munich, pp 707–713 (Recent advances in studies on cardiac structure and metabolism, vol 1)

Ravens KG (1970) Der Einfluß von anabolen Hormonen und von Diät auf den myokardialen Gehalt an energiereichen Phosphaten während der Infarktheilung. Verh Dtsch Ges Kreislaufforsch 36:314–319

Remes K, Kuoppasalmi K, Adlercreutz H (1979) Effect of long-term physical training on plasma testosterone, androstenedione, luteinizing hormone, and sex-hormone-binding globulin capacity. Scand J Clin Lab Invest 39:743–749

Rose RM, Bourne P, Poe RO, Mougey EH, Collins DR, Mason JW (1969) Androgen responses to stress. Psychosom Med 31/5:418–436

Schumann H (1939) Der Einfluß der männlichen Sexualhormone auf den Glykogen-, Phosagen- und Adenylpyrophosphatgehalt des Herzmuskels. Klin Wochenschr 18:925–927

Seliverstov SA (1969) The effect of nerobolon on the blood supply, cardiac activity, and haemodynamics. Farmakol Toksikol 32:59–62

Seyle H (1969) La evolution del concepto del stress. Folia Clin Int 32:471–489

Selye H (1970a) Experimental cardiovascular diseases, vol 2. Springer, Berlin Heidelberg New York

Selye H (1970b) Stress and ageing. Am Geriatr Soc 18:679–680

Shafrir E, Steinberg D (1960) The essential role of the adrenal cortex in the response of plasma free fatty acids, cholesterol, and phospholipids to epinephrine injection. J Clin Invest 39:310–319

Shillingford JP, Joplin CF, Jamieson CW, Rubens R (1980) Visit to Dr. Møller's clinic. Bull EOCCD 6

Short D (1977) The great circulatory paradox. Lancet I:1244–1247

Sobel H, Marmorston J (1958) Hormonal influences upon connective tissue's changes of aging. In: Pincus G (ed) Recent progress in hormone research, vol 14. Academic, New York

Starnes JW, Beyer RE, Edington DW (1981) Effects of age and cardiac work in vitro on mitochondrial oxidative phosphorylation and ($^3$H)-leucine incorporation. J Gerontol 36:130–135

Steffney M (1983) Relatively larger heart in children than in adults (in Danish). Politiken 5 Aug 1983

Stryer L (1975) Biochemistry. Freeman, San Francisco

Sufin G, Prutkin L (1974) Experimental diabetes and the response of the sex accessory organs of the castrate male rat to testosterone propinate. Invest Urol 11/5:361–369

Tainter ML, Arnold A, Beyler AL, Potts GO, Roth CH (1964) Anabolic steroids in the management of the diabetic patient. NY State J Med 64:1001–1009

Talaat M, Habib YA, Habib M (1957) The effect of testosterone on the carbohydrate metabolism in normal subjects. Arch Int Pharmacodyn 111/2:215–226

Talaat M, Habib YA, Hanna T (1958) Effect of testosterone propionate on the carbohydrate metabolism in the liver and muscle of male rabbits. Arch Int Pharmacodyn 116:410–417

Talaat M, Habib YA, Malek AY (1964) Effect of testosterone propionate on the carbohydrate metabolism in castrated male rabbits. Arch Int Pharmacodyn 151:369–382

Thaysen JH, Christensen LK, Kjerulf K (eds) (1975) Medicinsk kompendium, 11th edn. Nyt Nordisk, Copenhagen

Tsushima M (1975) Primary prevention of atherosclerotic vascular disease with ethylnandrol. Jpn Circ J 39/3:285–292

Tweedle D, Walton C, Johnston IDA (1973) The effect of an anabolic steroid on postoperative nitrogen balance. Br J Clin Pract 27/4:130–132

Urbanová D, Janda J, Mrhová O, Linhart J (1974) Enzyme changes in the ischemia of skeletal muscle and the effect of physical conditioning. A histochemical study. Histochem J 6:147–155

U.S. Diabetes Source Book (1969)

Vaissmann I, Cantisano L, Granato PO (1960) Über die blutcholesterolsenkende Wirkung androgener Hormone. Ärztl Forsch 15:530–534

Veil WH, Lippross O (1938) „Unspezifische" Wirkungen der männlichen Keimdrüsenhormone. Klin Wochenschr 17:615–627

Wagner H, Zierden E, Böckel K, Hauss WH (1975) Correlations between lipid and carbohydrate metabolism and testosterone serum levels in patients with myocardial infarction. Acta Endocrinol (Copenh) [Suppl] 199:425

Walker LD, Davidson JF, Young P, Conkie JA (1975) Plasma fibrinolytic activity following oral anabolic steroid therapy. Thromb Diathes Haemorrh 34:236–245

Weissel W (1962) Anaboles Hormon bei malignem oder kompliziertem Diabetes mellitus. Wien Klin Wochenschr 74:234–236

Weiner N (1980) Norepinephrine, epinephrine and the sympathomimetic amines. In: Gillman AG, Goodman LS, Gilman A (eds) Goodman and Gilman's the pharmacological basis of therapeutics, 6th edn. McMillan, New York, chap 8

Winther O (1965) Testosterone and fibrinolytic activity. Scand J Clin Lab Invest [Suppl] 99:207–210
Winther O (1966) Exercise and blood-fibrinolysis. Lancet I:1195–1196
World Health Organization (1972) Prevention of ischaemic heart disease. Metabolic aspects. WHO-Symposium, Madrid, 1972, WHO/CVD/73:3
Yarnell J (1980) Visit to Prof. Møller's clinic, Copenhagen. Bull EOCCD 6
Zetterquist S (1970) The effect of active training on the nutritive blood flow in exercising ischemic legs. J Clin Lab Invest 25:101–111

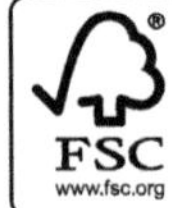

MIX
Papier aus verantwortungsvollen Quellen
Paper from responsible sources
FSC® C105338

If you have any concerns about our products,
you can contact us on
ProductSafety@springernature.com

In case Publisher is established outside the EU,
the EU authorized representative is:
Springer Nature Customer Service Center GmbH
Europaplatz 3, 69115 Heidelberg, Germany

Printed by Libri Plureos GmbH
in Hamburg, Germany